'This book will fill the gap between Western diving medicine and the acupuncture point of view. Also easy to access for non-acupuncture medicals.'

– *Menno TW Gaastra, M.D., medical director DAN Europe for the Netherlands*

'Janneke Vermeulen's book embodies both art and science – with her exquisite colour diving photographs, medical illustrations, and Western and Chinese medicine treatments, for ear, nose and throat (ENT) imbalances and other syndromes. The protocols are well organized, and can also be utilized for ENT problems caused by "frequent flying", chronic sinus issues, colds, etc. Her last chapter beautifully addresses the spirit and the receptive, yin aspect of the Water element, which encourages meditation and a sense of being present in the eternal Now.'

– *Mary Elizabeth Wakefield, L. Ac., M.S., M.M., Dipl. Ac., NCCAOM, author, international teacher of facial acupuncture and opera singer*

'Divers around the world should rejoice in seeing this book published. It is a comprehensive manual of health conditions associated with diving. Incorporating both Western and Chinese medicine perspectives, Janneke Vermeulen details the clinical features of disorders that can be aggravated or initiated by diving, or inhibit one's ability to enter the water in the first place. She gives numerous practical and effective treatments, acupuncture point combinations and lifestyle recommendations that will help practitioners treat divers better so that they can keep on diving.'

– *Lillian Pearl Bridges, author of* Face Reading in Chinese Medicine, 2nd Edition

DIVING MEDICAL ACUPUNCTURE

of related interest

The Living Needle
Modern Acupuncture Technique
Justin Phillips
ISBN 978 1 84819 381 9
eISBN 978 0 85701 339 2

Neuropuncture
A Clinical Handbook of Neuroscience Acupuncture, Second Edition
Michael D. Corradino
Foreword by Giovanni Maciocia
ISBN 978 1 84819 331 4
eISBN 978 0 85701 287 6

The Fundamentals of Acupuncture
Nigel Ching
Foreword by Charles Buck
ISBN 978 1 84819 313 0
eISBN 978 0 85701 266 1

The Yellow Monkey Emperor's Classic of Chinese Medicine
Damo Mitchell and Spencer Hill
ISBN 978 1 84819 286 7
eISBN 978 0 85701 233 3

DIVING MEDICAL ACUPUNCTURE

潜水和医疗针灸

Treatment and Prevention of Diving Medical Problems with a Focus on ENT Disorders

JANNEKE VERMEULEN

FOREWORD BY WILLIAM MACLEAN

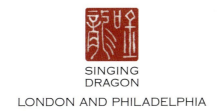

SINGING DRAGON

LONDON AND PHILADELPHIA

All medical illustrations © DNA Illustrations, Inc., www.dnaillustrations.com
Figure 1.1.5 and 4.1.1 used with permission of Lars Behnke.
Figure 1.1.6 used with permission of Francine Kreiss.
Figure 1.1.7 by Utagawa Yoshiiku (1864), copyright MFA, Boston, USA. Used with permission.
Figure 1.11.1a and 1.11.1b used with kind permission of Terry Oleson.
Figure 1.12.3 used with permission of Dr Simon Mitchell.
Figure 2.2.4 from Baguley (2000) used with permission of Oxford University Press.
Figure 7.2.1 by Katsushika Hokusai copyright Rijksmuseum
Amsterdam, the Netherlands. Used with permission.

First published in 2018
by Jessica Kingsley Publishers
73 Collier Street
London N1 9BE, UK
and
400 Market Street, Suite 400
Philadelphia, PA 19106, USA

www.jkp.com

Copyright © Janneke Vermeulen 2018
Foreword copyright © William Maclean 2018

Front cover image source: Shutterstock®.

All rights reserved. No part of this publication may be reproduced in any material form (including photocopying, storing in any medium by electronic means or transmitting) without the written permission of the copyright owner except in accordance with the provisions of the law or under terms of a licence issued in the UK by the Copyright Licensing Agency Ltd. www.cla.co.uk or in overseas territories by the relevant reproduction rights organization, for details see www.ifrro.org. Applications for the copyright owner's written permission to reproduce any part of this publication should be addressed to the publisher.

All sections marked with ⊕ can be downloaded at www.jkp.com/voucher for personal use with this programme, but may not be reproduced for any other purposes without the permission of the publisher.

Warning: The doing of an unauthorized act in relation to a copyright work may result in both a civil claim for damages and criminal prosecution.

Library of Congress Cataloging in Publication Data
A CIP catalog record for this book is available from the Library of Congress

British Library Cataloguing in Publication Data
A CIP catalogue record for this book is available from the British Library

ISBN 978 1 84819 323 9
eISBN 978 0 85701 276 0

Printed and bound in China

> The accompanying PDF can be downloaded from
> www.jkp.com/voucher using the code meHG2z8x

Contents

FOREWORD BY WILLIAM MACLEAN 9

Preface 11

Acknowledgements 17

1. EAR, NOSE AND THROAT DISORDERS. 21
耳鼻喉疾患

    1.1 Introduction 21

    1.2 Anatomy of the Ear 34
        局部解剖

    1.3 Anatomy of the Nose and Sinuses 36
        鼻和鼻窦的解剖

    1.4 Techniques for Clearing the Ears 38
        清洁中耳道的操作

    1.5 Disorders That May Cause Equalizing Problems 44
        可能导致平衡障碍的疾患

    1.6 Common Cold 53
        感冒

    1.7 Rhinosinusitis 68
        鼻窦炎

    1.8 Allergic Rhinitis and Non-Allergic Rhinitis 95
        过敏性鼻炎

    1.9 Otitis 108
        耳炎

    1.10 Surfer's Ear 119
        冲浪耳

    1.11 Perforation of the Tympanic Membrane 121
        鼓膜穿孔

    1.12 Tinnitus 124
        耳鸣

2. **TEMPOROMANDIBULAR JOINT DISORDERS** 143
   颞下颌关节疾患

   2.1 Temporomandibular Joint Disorder and the Regulator 143
   颞下颌关节疾患和调节器

   2.2 Temporomandibular Joint Disorder and Tinnitus. 144
   颞下颌关节疾患和耳鸣

   2.3 Muscles and Ligaments of the TMJ and Middle Ear 152
   和中耳的肌肉和肌腱

   2.4 TMJ Disorders 157
   颞下颌关节疾患

3. **SEASICKNESS** 171
   晕动病

   3.1 Introduction 171

4. **DECOMPRESSION ILLNESS** 177
   减压病

   4.1 The Onset of Decompression Illness 177
   减压病的发生

5. **DIVING, MEDICATION AND NATURAL STIMULANTS** 186
   潜水 药物和天然兴奋剂

   5.1 Medication, Side-Effects and Contraindications for Diving. . . . 186
   潜水用药 副作用和禁忌症

   5.2 Diving and Migraine 188
   潜水和偏头痛

   5.3 Diving and Hypertension. 194
   潜水和高血压

   5.4 Natural Stimulants 199
   天然兴奋剂

6. **ADDITIONAL INFORMATION AND ADVICE REGARDING DIVING-RELATED DISORDERS** 202
   与潜水有关的附加资料和建议

   6.1 Introduction 202

   6.2 Neck and Back Disorders. 202
   颈和腰部疾患

   6.3 Muscle Disorders 213
   肌肉的疾患

   6.4 Lung Disorders. 215
   肺的疾患

6.5 Heart Disorders 218
心的疾患

6.6 Digestive Disorders 221
消化疾患

6.7 Stress and Panic 222
压力和惊慌

7. **DIVING AND MEDITATION** **228**
潜水与冥想

   7.1 Introduction 228

   7.2 Meditation and Flotation 228
   冥想与漂浮

   7.3 Flotation Tank 229
   漂浮罐

   7.4 Brain Waves 230
   脑电波

CONCLUSION **232**

Appendix I: Glossary of Terminology 233

*Appendix II: Acupuncture Points with
Specific ENT and TMJ Actions* 235

*Appendix III: Acupuncture Points with
Specific ENT- and TMJ-Related Indications* 240

FOREWORD

Chinese medicine is a wonderfully elastic system of medicine, capable of innovation in areas beyond the imaginings of its ancient architects. Acupuncture in particular has infiltrated the medical mainstream, finding its way into the armoury of orthopaedics, gynaecology and dentistry. Now its scope is expanding further, reaching into the oceans and lakes of the world.

The first time I donned a regulator and wetsuit to dive the crystalline waters of the Red Sea, a rich and hitherto unknown world opened up. Exploring Turkish wrecks, meeting hammerheads, barracuda and pilot whales while floating, weightless, through the lavish reef, I was hooked. Many years and many dives later, having experienced the highs and lows of the underwater world, I know that access to the watery realm can be all too easily denied by the challenges that being submerged presents to the land dweller.

It's the simple things that make for a great or difficult dive experience. An ideal location with superlative visibility can be ruined by seasickness, congested Eustachian tubes or blocked sinuses. An inability to equalize pressure in the middle ear can lead to pain or even rupture of the eardrum, or derail access to the dive site if flying is required. Having a means to address these problems effectively (and often immediately), without resorting to medication, is the holy grail of the diving physician. With *Diving Medical Acupuncture*, Janneke has amply demonstrated the significant role the acupuncturist can have in keeping divers in the water. Her approach is based on experience as a PADI[1] Divemaster and this shows in her understanding of the practical realities of the dive itself, the potential problems that can mar the experience, and the effective solutions to be found in the Chinese medical approach. Each section combines a clear discussion of the relevant anatomy and pathology, augmented by splendid illustrations to enhance understanding. The pluses and minuses of mainstream medical treatment

---
1 Professional Association of Diving Instructors.

are discussed, along with appropriate Chinese medical pattern differentiation that focuses on those areas in which the Chinese medicine approach really shines, and Janneke does a first-rate job of linking the two systems of thought and producing practical and easily implemented strategies. As an immediate and portable skill, acupuncture can be applied at the dive site without resorting to potentially complicating medications. For more persistent or recurrent problems, proven treatments applied in a professional setting can often correct even the most recalcitrant problems and return divers to the water.

Diving Medical Acupuncture is thoroughly researched and referenced, and fills a much-needed niche in the expanding repertoire of effective Chinese medical therapy. This practical book will find an appreciative readership in divers and their therapists, and an equally enthusiastic following among practitioners dealing with ear, nose and throat issues commonly seen in general practice.

William Maclean, practitioner of Chinese medicine and author of
the *Clinical Handbook of Internal Medicine, Clinical Manual of Chinese
Herbal Patent Medicines* and *Clinical Handbook of Chinese Herbs*

Preface

As a passionate diving acupuncturist, I have written this book for all my acupuncturist colleagues around the globe who want to treat divers with specific diving medical problems in the most profound way. It is also for physicians to gain more knowledge about diving medicine and to clarify possible treatments from the Western and Chinese viewpoints. This book contains practical advice as well, which you as a professional can give to the diver who consults you and which naturally can be used independently by the diver.

Because about 70 per cent of all diving medical problems are ENT (ear, nose and throat) related, the biggest part of the book deals with that. My intention is to contribute to the understanding of ENT disorders, their treatment in general and how these disorders are often related to changes in ambient pressure, such as can occur when diving or flying. Interactions between pressure change and the air-filled cavities of the body applies equally to aviation as well as diving, and the same acupuncture treatments are suitable for aviation-related medical problems.

The main difference regarding ENT disorders seen with divers compared to ENT disorders in general is the consequence of being submerged and having to deal with the hydrostatic pressure that interacts with our body and mind. The importance of well-functioning ENT structures is illustrated clearly by pressure changes in a way that will contribute to more understanding of ENT disorders in general.

Having divers in your acupuncture practice implies that you need to have certain knowledge about Western diving medicine, diving physics, diving techniques and Chinese medicine.

This book will give useful insights to treating divers with acupuncture, resulting in more diving comfort, diving safety, diving pleasure and better general health. The medical illustrations in this book take you into the depth of the body, to make physical structures more clear and to help you understand better which parts are affected when we needle acupuncture points. The underwater photos bring you into the depth of the ocean to show you the hidden magic, as that is the reason a diver wants to get rid of annoying ENT disorders and go back there. So let me take you on an adventurous journey and make an unknown world known.

In around 300 BCE Aristotle was the first physician to describe perforation of the tympanic membrane in divers. This ancient medical description concretizes that diving, diving medicine and equalizing problems have a long history. Luckily nowadays we have a lot of more information about the ENT structures and appropriate knowledge to prevent this painful – and very dangerous when underwater – medical condition. It has become clear that acupuncture can contribute to its prevention.

To me, diving is a fantastic way to enjoy one of the beauties the planet has given us. Being a part of the magnificent underwater world for a certain time is almost an addiction. The feeling of oneness with the surroundings and experiencing the almost complete silence is unique. The only sound there is comes from the bubbles from your regulator. Watching thousands and thousands of small colourful fish close to the coral reefs, a fascinating whale shark recognizable by its white speckles, swift manta rays, a lovely turtle swimming to the water surface to get some air, being *out of the blue* (as we call diving in totally blue underwater surroundings) *and* the sparkling sunbeams of the early morning reflecting in the water give me a feeling of intense happiness. Diving makes me feel serene, clear and completely balanced.

In this book I write about my treatments, which I have performed since 2003 when I started diving myself. This book is focused on which acupuncture points and which combination of points give the best results when treating diving medical problems. For instance, combining Chinese acupuncture with Japanese Yamamoto New Scalp Acupuncture (YNSA), gives a very strong and positive effect on many disorders in the ENT regions. I will explain some important diving techniques and give information about physical and mental aspects: details you just don't know when you have had no diving education. My intention is that you will be able to imagine how it is to be a part of the underwater world, which complaints are most common, why they happen and what you can do to affect them positively.

The main focus is on ENT disorders because clearing the ears is the most commonly experienced problem for divers. This specific equalizing problem is the number-one problem in aviation as well.

To give a clear and comprehensive picture I have added a summary of Western medical treatment for each disorder, because the combination of Western and Chinese medicine is necessary to understand the medical conditions and treatment options in the most profound way. For me Western and Chinese medicine are like an oyster shell. Just like the parts of this symmetrical bivalve, the insights from both sciences can be placed exactly upon each other and form one solid unit with the pearl of wisdom and integrated knowledge inside.

For each disorder I have supplied a concise Chinese medical pattern differentiation to provide an overview of the most common causes of the disorders.

I have added the Chinese names for the acupuncture points in addition to the English numbering. In the appendices I have included the English translation of these names as well because they give good insights into the actions of the points. I offer an extended point selection for each complaint because it is good to be informed as broadly as possible and it gives you more treatment options. It is good to bring some variety in your treatment so no habituation can occur; also, when a complaint is very hard to influence it's advisable to try another point selection or add some extra points.

With respect to the actions of the acupuncture points regarding the specific condition I have supplied a concise picture to keep the book user friendly. An overview of all actions of and indications for the acupuncture points that influence ENT and TMJ (temporomandibular joint) disorders is given in two appendices at the back of this book. In the main text (in the 'Explanation' sections) I have added some of the most important indications to provide a clear and more illuminating ENT vision.

For clarity, both the Chinese names and their translations are given for the various qualities of the pulses.

Regarding Chinese medical terminology, I have used the Pinyin names to stay as close as possible to the origin of (and the original meaning in) Chinese medicine for the Vital Substances such as Jing, Shen, Xue, Jin Ye and Wei Qi. A compact and simplified glossary is included in the back of the book (see Table AI.1). I have capitalized the Pinyin names so that they show up obviously in the text, and also technical terms like Wind-Cold, Heat, Spleen, Kidney, Dampness and Phlegm to distinguish them clearly from Western medical terminology.

For completeness I have added practical advice for the diver for each medical issue. This advice gives acupuncturists a better understanding of what diving involves and the acupuncturist will be able to give clear advice to the diver. With all this information I want to make an unknown world known because the more understanding there is about diving the better the diving medical problems can be treated.

In general the sections covering the diving medical problems are structured as follows:

1. Western medicine (definition and aetiology, diagnosis, treatment and the side-effects of medication).

2. Chinese medicine (definition and aetiology, pattern differentiation, treatment principle, and the specific selection of acupuncture points with explanation and clinical notes).

3. Advice for the diver.

> The advice for the diver sections are available to download from www.jkp.com/voucher using the code meHG2z8x

With this book I am offering a comprehensive overall picture to handle and treat the most common diving medical problems by means of acupuncture. I expect this clinical manual will be helpful in giving essential information to keep divers diving in a safe and healthy way and extending your ENT knowledge in general.

Acupuncture already improves the quality of diving just by working on the diver's general health. For example, when you tonify Lung-Qi and promote its descending and diffusing, the diver will be able to breathe more deeply and in a more relaxed way. This results in using less of the compressed air from the tank and having more time to stay under water. The diver will be very grateful for that!

Besides the existing complaints a diver can have, it can be good anyway to undergo some treatments once in a while or before a diving holiday to support general health.

My clinical experience is based on working in my own practice with acupuncture, Chinese herbal medicine, Chinese facial diagnostics and physiotherapy in The Hague, the Netherlands, since 1994. I have been studying Chinese medicine for years in Europe, the USA and China and am inspired by Yamamoto New Scalp Acupuncture (YNSA). At the International Acupuncture Training Centre in Beijing (2004), where I wanted to gain more knowledge about ENT disorders to improve my diving medical treatments, the doctors thought it was weird to practise diving: 'Why do you go under water and *watch* fish? We *eat* them...'

I am privileged as an acupuncturist/physiotherapist to have had, as an exception, the opportunity to attended several ENT-related diving medicine courses with the Scott Haldane Foundation. The Scott Haldane Foundation is an international institute dedicated to education of physicians in diving and hyperbaric medicine worldwide. Besides my (para) medical background I have trained as a PADI Divemaster.

The knowledge gained from all the above is fundamental to this book. Most of the diving medical knowledge in this book is based on what I have learned during my diving medicine courses and my own diving experiences. In addition, I have used the book '*Duikgeneeskunde, Theorie en Praktijk*, tweede druk' (*Diving Medicine, second edition*) by J.J. Brandt Corstius, S.M. Dermout and L. Feenstra,[1] and

---

1 Brandt Corstius, J.J., Dermout, S.M. and Feenstra, L., *Duikgeneeskunde, Theorie en Praktijk*, tweede druk, Elsevier, Amsterdam, 2007.

my own acupuncture expertise has been supplemented by the *Clinical Handbook of Internal Medicine*, Volumes 1, 2 and 3, by William Maclean and Jane Lyttleton.[2]

For describing the actions of the acupuncture points in a consistent and international way, I have used terminology from *A Manual of Acupuncture* by Peter Deadman and Mazin Al-Khafajin with Kevin Baker.[3] To offer the most extensive insights and applications, the actions themselves have been complemented – where of interest – with information from *Tekstboek Acupunctuur, deel I, Punten* (Textbook of Acupuncture, Part I, Points) from physician Walter Boermeester,[4] and *The Foundations of Chinese Medicine: A Comprehensive Text*, third edition and *De Grondslagen van de Chinese Geneeskunde, Een Complete Basishandleiding voor Acupuncturisten en Fytotherapeuten, Tweede Uitgave* (*The Foundations of Chinese Medicine: A Complete Basic Manual for Acupuncturists and Herbalists, second edition*) from Giovanni Maciocia.[5] I have also used these books to compile the list of indications in Appendix III.

The medical English terminology regarding arteries, nerves, muscles and their functions conforms with *Gray's Anatomy for Students*, third edition (Churchill Livingstone: Elsevier, 2015) from Richard L. Drake, A. Wayne Vogle and Adam W.M. Mitchell,[6] who follow the 'Terminologia Anatomica'[7] in the interest of uniformity.

The idea of treating divers in my practice was born in 2003 after one of my patients asked if I could treat her equalizing problem, which occurred every third day of all her diving holidays. This problem resulted in not being able to dive any more and having to stay on deck of the boat. My treatment was focused on transforming Phlegm, addressing the underlying deficiencies, and opening the nose, Eustachian tube and sinuses. After some acupuncture treatments and a diving week in Egypt she came back to the practice happy, telling me she didn't experience any ear problem at all and was able to dive every day! I was also triggered by all the magic underwater stories from another diving patient. Having my own special memory of snorkelling once at Koh Samet in Thailand I decided to get my diving licence. I started with the NOB Open Water and

---

2   Maclean, W. and Lyttleton, J., *Clinical Handbook of Internal Medicine*, Volume 1, fifth printing, University of Western Sydney, Sydney, 2008; *Clinical Handbook of Internal Medicine*, Volume 2, second printing, University of Western Sydney, Sydney, 2003; *Clinical Handbook of Internal Medicine*, Volume 3, second printing, Pangolin Press, Waverley, 2013.

3   Deadman, P., Al-Khafaji, M. and Baker, K., *A Manual of Acupuncture*, Journal of Chinese Medicine Publications, Hove, 2015.

4   Boermeester, W., *Tekstboek Acupunctuur, deel I, Punten*, Chinese Medicine Data, Kapellen, 1989.

5   Maciocia, G., *The Foundations of Chinese Medicine: A Comprehensive Text*, third edition, Elsevier, Amsterdam, 2015; *De Grondslagen van de Chinese Geneeskunde, Een Complete Basishandleiding voor Acupuncturisten en Fytotherapeuten, Tweede Uitgave*, Churchill Livingstone, New York, 2005.

6   Drake, R.L., Wayne Vogle, A. and Adam Mitchell, A.W.M., *Gray's Anatomy for Students*, third edition, Churchill Livingstone, Edinburgh, 2015.

7   Federative Committee on Anatomical Terminology, *Terminologia Anatomica: International Anatomical Terminology*, second edition, Thieme, Stuttgart, 2011.

Advanced licences (I was sold after the first lesson in a swimming pool) and since 2005 I have had the PADI Divemaster licence.

During my diving lessons and first two diving holidays in Egypt and at Bonaire, it became clear to me that *clearing the ears* is a common problem seen with divers. I even needled one of the instructors before a required dive for my PADI Advanced licence in the Caribbean Sea, who suddenly developed a common cold. With needles in his face he tested my diving homework and meanwhile his nose opened. After that he guided me without problems during a compass dive in the shallow water close to the harbour of Kralendijk.

With a leaflet titled 'Diving without problems with acupuncture' and an interview, 'Acupuncture for Divers', in the Dutch *Diving Magazine* (Magazine Duiken) in May 2004 in the Netherlands the specialism *Diving Medical Acupuncture* was established!

Not everyone will be able to have the privilege of studying Western diving medicine, as diving medicine belongs to the field of the Western physician, or be able to experience what diving is. That's why I hope this book will be a guide to help my colleagues everywhere around the globe to treat specific diving medical problems optimally.

I had to walk a long path to create this first Chinese diving medicine book, developed in spare hours in my practice work, and most came from recalling what I had learned in the previous years. There was so much information in my head about so many different disciplines, details, facts and insights. It took time and effort to let it come out, to structure it clearly, and to present it all as concisely as possible in one practical book. But here it is: the pearl of integrated diving medicine that came out of the oyster!

Acknowledgements

When writing a medical book – especially in a foreign language – you need support in all ways because it is a very comprehensive and prolonged project. I am grateful for all kinds of contributions from so many wonderful people from every corner of this globe!

First, I want to thank my friend Lillian Pearl Bridges from Seattle – the world's leading expert in Chinese face reading and diagnosis – from the bottom of my heart for encouraging me to write this book. Lillian supported me with confidence while I was searching for a clear structure and a complete set of medical topics for my book. Taking the photographs for Lillian's second edition of *Face Reading in Chinese Medicine,* and working long days together to get them ready for her publisher, Elsevier, was a challenge as I developed as a photographer and face reader at the same time. Lillian, thank you so much for inspiring me to use the writer genes I have inherited from my grandfather, J.J.C. Böckling, and my mother, Annemiek Böckling, both authors of several books.

Second, I have more than thousands thanks for William Maclean from Australia, practitioner of Chinese medicine, author of the *Clinical Handbook of Internal Medicine, Clinical Manual of Chinese Herbal Patent Medicines* and *Clinical Handbook of Chinese Herbs* and, just like me, a keen diver. He was a fantastic mentor in helping me make my first book appropriate for both an international and an academic audience, with consistent terminology. William let me see my script through the eyes of a professional author, and his advice has contributed to a compact and user-friendly book.

Many thanks to Mary Elizabeth Wakefield from New York, acupuncturist, international teacher in Constitutional Facial Acupuncture and friend, who supported me with humour and wisdom while writing. In the beginning when I was making sustained progress, she told me, 'Janneke, don't count the pages, just write!' Later, when I was working on a difficult format change, we phoned and I said almost desperately, 'I can hang that book in a tree.' Mary's response was, 'Oh Janneke, you are so funny, hanging a book in a tree…and the birds will do the rest for you!' The laughter gave me energy to continue the hard work.

Mary's first book, *Constitutional Facial Acupuncture*, was my second project as a photographer.

Alexandra and David Baker from North Carolina: thank you for the wonderful illustrations. This complete set of very specific subjects shows exactly what I am expressing in words and they contribute to more understanding. Thanks for the original, colourful and scientific look!

Vielen Dank Lars Behnke from Germany, full-stack developer, biologist and diver, thank you for allowing me to use clear illustrations of hand signals from your book and mobile application *SCUBA Diving Hand Signals*.

Thank you Terry Oleson from Los Angeles, acupuncturist and author of *Auriculotherapy Manual*, for letting me use one of your ear illustrations in an adapted way in my book!

Thanks to my herbal teacher Yifan Yang, acupuncturist and author of *Chinese Herbal Medicines* and *Chinese Herbal Formulas* for providing the needed Chinese characters used to the subjects and sections of the chapters and all your personal support: *xièxie nǐ*. Thank you Zhigang Yang, my other Chinese herbal teacher, for discussing several Chinese medical topics.

Also thanks to Virginia Doran, acupuncturist and international teacher of Facial Rejuvenation Acupuncture from New York, who gave me good practical advice relating to the focus of my book.

Many thanks to Menno Gaastra, diving physician in the Netherlands, for reviewing the Western diving medical parts of my book script in the final stage. Thanks to Judith Rietveld, head editor of *Magazine Duiken*, for your support in many ways.

Thanks to my friends Betty Mouzo Gonzales and Bajah Freeman, acupuncturists in the Netherlands, for giving me clear and grounded feedback as well as positive criticism while working on this book, and always being willing to discuss and debate parts of the book. Jacqueline Sander, Western physician and friend in the Netherlands, thank you for supporting me by checking the illustrations during the book's development. Individual educational supervisor and friend Ineke Geneste, thanks for your advice regarding source references.

Thanks to physician and acupuncturist Akeel Qureshi, and Pauline Hulspas, industrial psychologist/diving instructor (who trained me to become a PADI Divemaster in 2006) in the Netherlands, for critiquing the book script.

Thank you CT Holman, acupuncturist from Redwood Spring, Portland, for being enthusiastic about my book from the beginning, always making time for answering my questions and advising me on background literature when needed.

Many thanks also to international colleagues and friends for advising and thinking with me about certain parts of the book: Rik Lim from New York, Heidi-Anna Grüber from Austria, Katherine Andersen from Durengo, Colorado, and Patricia Gust from St Paul, Minnesota.

ACKNOWLEDGEMENTS

Thank you Meindert van Rumpt, orofacial physical therapist in the Netherlands, for evaluating the chapter about TMJ disorders.

Many thanks to Jan-Jaap Brandt Corstius, exercise physiologist and active in diving and hyperbaric medicine, and Sylvia Dermout, gynaecologist and diving physician, from the Netherlands for the unique chance you have given me to expand my diving medical knowledge at the highest level possible. Without this, this book wouldn't be here!

A big warm thank you to Gerard Smienk, acupuncturist and one of the directors of the institute TCM Postgraduate in the Netherlands, who organized my first official teaching day about acupuncture for ENT disorders seen with divers in Amsterdam on 20 November 2015.

Many thanks to my diving and non-diving patients who have supported me non-stop and with lots of interest during my writing process.

I want to thank Jessica Kingsley, chairman and managing director of Singing Dragon and Jessica Kingsley Publishers, for having faith in my innovative book, for being the editor for it and giving me the chance to show my work to the world. Claire Wilson, senior commissioning editor, thank you for the inspirational talk we had about my book plan at the Pacific Conference in San Diego (2010), when you were working for Elsevier, and for your assistance after joining JKP, triggering Jessica to read the submitted script later in 2015. Victoria Peters, production manager, and Hannah Snetsinger, editorial assistant, thanks for all your clear advice while finishing my book.

Thank you Bas, my eldest brother, for supporting me with the illustrations. Thanks to my sister Caroline for telling me without doubt that this book will be a best seller when I was struggling during the writing process, and my youngest brother Pieter for believing in my work at all times.

Also thanks to my dear nephews and nieces who encouraged me cheerfully during this writing process!

And last but not least. This book is dedicated to my dear parents for supporting me in the way I needed it and to my grandfather, J.J.C. Böckling, called *Apa*. Apa would have been proud that the writer's baton has been passed.

••• CHAPTER 1 •••

EAR, NOSE AND THROAT DISORDERS

耳鼻喉疾患

1.1 INTRODUCTION

What is more frustrating than being packed into your diving suit, getting just below the water surface in a spectacular tropical ocean, seeing beautiful corals and colourful fish down under and finding out that one of your ears is not cooperating as you go down, feeling a painful pressure in it that you can't get rid of, and even ascending a little doesn't help?

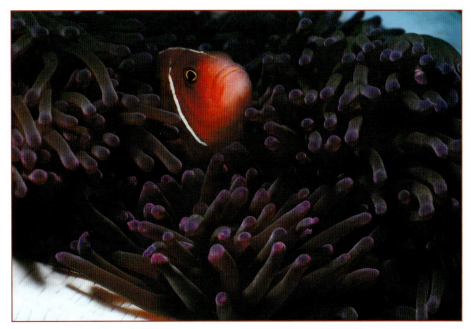

Figure 1.1.1 Under the water surface a fairytale is waiting
Photo: Janneke Vermeulen, Bohol Island, the Philippines, 2008

The most common problem experienced by divers is not being able to clear the ears or having difficulty equalizing. Clearing the ears is also called *ear clearing* or *pressure equalization* and means *the equalization of pressure in the middle ears caused by the ambient pressure*. No or insufficient equalization means that diving isn't possible, or that the diver has to discontinue the dive he or she is making.

Ears are essential for the human being. When working well, they give us lots of information about the outside world and they affect our equilibrium. When hearing less, nothing, buzzing, sizzling, ringing or dealing with vertigo, life can be influenced by it enormously. Caring for ears correctly is of great importance for their good functioning and thereby for quality of life.

The ear is a very sensitive organ and by no means built for being under water like the ears of a shark. Maybe you are even surprised to discover that the shark has ears but this cartilaginous fish has! There is a small hole on each side of the shark's head, just behind the eyes, named the *endolymphatic pore*. This pore is connected directly to the inner ear by an endolymphatic duct. The inner ear of a shark, like the human ear, can perceive sound, acceleration and gravity. The shark is especially allured by 'irregular, low-frequency vibrations (particularly 40Hz or below)'[1] and can detect sound from 'distances of more than a mile'.[2] The hearing range of a shark is 10–800Hz and of a human 25–16,000Hz.[3] Luckily the shark has no middle ear, otherwise this fish would have problems clearing the ears with the very short fins he has…

Clearing the ears is the first thing a diver has to learn and the first thing the diver has to do when bringing the head under water to start a dive. As, human beings, we have to adjust carefully to the surrounding when we are submerged, in particular when descending and ascending. The changing ambient pressure influences the position of the tympanic membrane, which has no function under water for hearing. Hearing only happens by skull bone conduction in this situation. Under water we hear about 30 per cent in comparison to above the water surface. Because there is no air conduction under water it's difficult for a human to determine the direction of sound. It seems as if sound is coming from *above*. Under water sound travels about 4.5 times faster than by air.

---

1   Springer, V.G. and Gold, J.P., *Sharks in Question: The Smithsonian Answer Book*, Smithsonian Institute Press, Washington, DC, 1989 (p.74).
2   Springer, V.G. and Gold, J.P., *Sharks in Question: The Smithsonian Answer Book*, Smithsonian Institute Press, Washington, DC, 1989 (p.74).
3   Smith, M.F.L., Warmolts, D., Thoney, D. and Hueter, R. (eds) *The Elasmobranch Husbandry Manual: Captive Care of Sharks, Rays, and Their Relatives*, Ohio Biological Survey, Columbus, OH, 2004.

EAR, NOSE AND THROAT DISORDERS

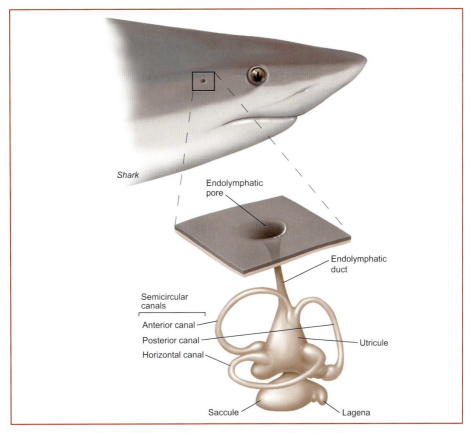

Figure 1.1.2 Why does a shark not need to clear its ears?

Ignoring signals such as pressure or pain in the ear can have big consequences, such as a rupture of the tympanic membrane, hearing loss or tinnitus. Divers sometimes have a tendency not to listen well to what their body tells them because they are in a holiday mood and everything is fun, and they are impressed by all the beautiful things they see around them. They go a lot deeper than scheduled to get a nice photo shot of a turtle that swims away to the depths, or even decide to go downwards again when performing the safety stop to finish the dive. And of course, the turtle is much quicker and impossible to catch up with! Or a diver may get nervous because the other divers are already deep down under and he or she wants to be with them to feel safe, so does not react on feeling a warning pressure in his or her ear(s).

Causes of Ear Equalization Problems

Problems with clearing the ears can be caused by factors such as:

- the common cold
- rhinosinusitis

- allergic rhinitis

- hyperreactivity of the mucosa in the nose and the Eustachian tube

- mechanical defects in the nose (for example septum deviation, polyps)

- wrongly performed clearing techniques (descending too quickly, descending with the head downwards or starting to clear the ears too late)[4]

- yo-yo actions while diving (repeatedly going up and down due to poor buoyancy control: the frequent pressure changes may irritate the mucous membranes in the Eustachian tube causing them to swell)[5]

- smoking[6]

- premenstrual oedema of the mucous membranes[7]

- stress (clamping on the regulator)[8]

- otitis

- a cerumen plug.

BOX 1.1.1 PRESSURE EQUALIZATION

Equalization of pressure implies: equalizing of under- or overpressure in the middle ears and sinuses caused by the ambient pressure. The sinuses clear automatically if there are no obstructions. While diving, the middle ears need to be equalized *actively during the descent* and usually clear automatically while ascending.

Treating Divers and Being a Diver

When treating and advising about problems with clearing the ears I believe that it is of indisputable importance to know what diving is, else you can't offer an optimal acupuncture treatment. You just can't compare diving with other sports like tennis or hockey. When diving, very specific disorders can occur

---

4 Brandt Corstius, J.J., Dermout, S.M. and Feenstra, L., *Duikgeneeskunde, Theorie en Praktijk*, tweede druk, Elsevier, Amsterdam, 2007.
5 Brandt Corstius, J.J., Dermout, S.M. and Feenstra, L., *Duikgeneeskunde, Theorie en Praktijk*, tweede druk, Elsevier, Amsterdam, 2007.
6 Brandt Corstius, J.J., Dermout, S.M. and Feenstra, L., *Duikgeneeskunde, Theorie en Praktijk*, tweede druk, Elsevier, Amsterdam, 2007.
7 Brandt Corstius, J.J., Dermout, S.M. and Feenstra, L., *Duikgeneeskunde, Theorie en Praktijk*, tweede druk, Elsevier, Amsterdam, 2007.
8 As observed in my own clinical experience.

due to the ambient pressure, such as nitrogen narcosis, oxygen intoxication and decompression illness.

When you treat divers the ideal situation is to be a diver yourself because diving has an extra dimension. When you dive you are part of another world. You are floating. You have to deal with the pressure from the water on your body. You are dependent on a tank filled with compressed air, giving you a limited time to stay in this world, which is not visible from the outside. This way of diving is called *scuba diving* (*scuba* means 'self-contained underwater breathing apparatus'). If you have never been under water with a *regulator* (a breathing machine), have never felt the pressure of the water on your body, you can't imagine well how these particular things interact with your body and mind. It is something to experience: the pressure in your ears, which increases when you descend (and you need to know how to diminish this pressure correctly) and the dry and cold air you breathe in through the regulator. This air can irritate the mucous membranes, resulting in a dry throat, and sometimes in hyperventilation, coughing, mucus production and some difficulty swallowing.

Non-divers don't usually think about the fact that when you are in tropical waters the corals are full of bacteria, which mainly arise when it is windy. On a windy day the waves move the water so the bacteria (divers call it *sediment*) eddy in the water, and visibility under water therefore is usually reduced. All those bacteria enter the external acoustic meatus and can cause serious problems. Lots of swimming pools – where many diving courses are given – are unfortunately sources of bacteria as well. There are specific ways to clean the ears after diving in open water or a swimming pool. It is important to perform these carefully to prevent otitis externa (see Section 1.9) after swimming and surfing likewise.

Types of Divers

In my practice I treat a lot of recreational divers, freedivers and professional divers with ENT disorders. The professionals include instructors, Divemasters, underwater photographers and sometimes divers who work under the water surface for hours repairing boats. For the professional divers it is essential to have no medical problems because diving is their job and income. Professional divers also include police divers, media divers (working for TV channels such as National Geographic or the BBC) and scientific divers. Besides the divers, I also see swimmers and surfers dealing with ear, nose and throat disorders.

BOX 1.1.2 SCIENTIFIC DIVERS

Worldwide, *scientific divers* (professional divers with a background of marine biology, marine chemistry, marine geology or marine physics) investigate the underwater environment. Scientific divers make movies and photographs of the underwater world, take biological, chemical or geological samples and study microsystems. Their research delivers essential information which reveals that a healthy marine life is necessary for our existence on earth. For example, the phytoplankton of the oceans produces about 50 per cent of our required oxygen supply![9] Coral reefs contribute to the development of medication against cancer, AIDS, asthma, arthritis and other inflammatory disorders as they contain powerful medical substances. Also the current killing of 100 million sharks per year (due to overfishing and bycatch) results in a disturbance of the total underwater ecosystem and damage to the coral reefs, which are important habitats for fish, sponges, algae, molluscs, turtles, and so on.

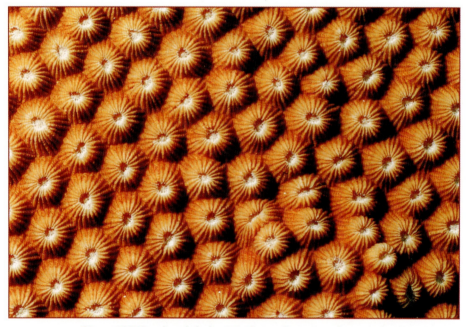

Figure 1.1.3 Coral reefs belong to the *underwater pharmacy*.
Corals (e.g. tunicates), algae, sponges and molluscs are used for medication against cancer, AIDS, asthma, arthritis and other inflammatory disorders
Photo: Janneke Vermeulen, Bohol Island, the Philippines, 2008

Luxury Problem?

Equalizing issues in divers may sound like a luxury problem but it by no means is. When you are unable to clear your ears you usually experience problems in normal life (i.e. above the water surface) as well, like having recurring common colds, chronic rhinosinusitis, otitis media, allergic or non-allergic rhinitis

---

9   National Research Council, *From Monsoons to Microbes: Understanding the Ocean's Role in Human Health*, The National Academies Press, Washington, DC, 1999.

combined with a low energy level: reasons enough to be treated anyway. When the diver is free of ear, nose and throat disorders equalization is in general no issue, as long as clearing techniques are performed correctly.

Diving Medical Examination

When diving it is strongly recommended that you have a medical examination by a diving physician to determine if you are *fit to dive* or not, because a diving medical examination may uncover issues you may not be aware of and which may be risky while diving (both Perth Scuba and PADI Asia Pacific give this advice). In the Netherlands, PADI and the NOB (Nederlandse Onderwatersport Bond) require a diving medical examination. The recommended frequency of the diving medical examination differs internationally from one to five years.

There are self-declaration forms (e.g. from PADI or the UK Diving Medical Committee) but if you answer just one question with yes, you should be examined by a diving medical physician. However, a questionnaire cannot estimate or explain the risks involved.

There are certain disorders that are absolute contraindications for diving, like having had a spontaneous pneumothorax, currently suffering from epilepsy, being pregnant or an acute otitis media. The use of certain medications, such as beta-blockers, anticoagulants and antidepressants, can be an absolute or relative contraindication for diving. When taking medication it is usually the underlying condition that can be the decisive reason for not being certified fit to dive, as well as the side-effects of the medication.

Ambient Pressure

Here is some general information to get a better picture about diving and the effects of the pressure of the water on our body:

- The most important diving law is *Boyle's Law*: The volume of a gas at constant temperature varies inversely with the pressure exerted on it.[10]

$$P \times V = C$$

This means: Pressure x Volume = Constant.

We use Boyle's law to measure air consumption at different depths and to determine the needed amount of air for a dive (the air consumption is based on 20 litres per minute at sea level). At sea level the ambient pressure is 1 ATA (atmosphere absolute – substantially equal

---

10 Brandt Corstius, J.J., Dermout, S.M. and Feenstra, L., *Duikgeneeskunde, Theorie en Praktijk*, tweede druk, Elsevier, Amsterdam, 2007.

to 1 bar). The *atmospheric pressure* is the pressure produced by the weight of atmospheric gases.

Every ten metres of water column gives the same pressure as the atmosphere (1 ATA). This pressure is called *hydrostatic pressure* and is produced by the weight of water, which increases with depth. This implies that at 10 metres depth we measure 2 ATA, at 20 metres it is 3 ATA, at 30 metres it's 4 ATA and so on. The deeper you go, the more influence there will be on your body due to the increased pressure.

The air-containing parts of the body, like the middle ear and the lungs, are pressed together when you descend and the degree of this depends on the ambient pressure (see Figure 1.1.4). In other words: the volume of air decreases and its density increases during the descent. When you ascend the air-filled cavities expand because the ambient pressure diminishes: the volume of air increases and its density decreases.

The air volume in your jacket decreases and increases likewise while descending and ascending. You need to regulate your buoyancy by increasing or decreasing the amount of air in your diving BCD (buoyancy control device) jacket with an inflator and deflator.

- To prevent decompression illness and barotrauma the recommended rate to ascend while scuba diving is ten metres per minute (average 9–12 metres).

- The maximum depth for recreational diving with compressed air according PADI[11] is 40 metres. Within this limit repetitive dives and normal ascents can be made safely. When diving deeper than 60 metres there is an unacceptable risk on oxygen intoxication.

---

11 PADI (the Professional Association Diving of Instructors) is the biggest diving organization on the globe.

EAR, NOSE AND THROAT DISORDERS

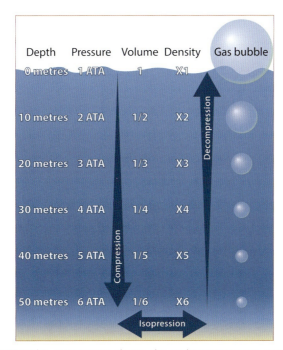

Figure 1.1.4 This ocean view shows the ambient pressure at sea level (0 m) and at various depths. The increase and decrease of ambient pressure has consequences for the volume of air and its density

Diving Hand Signals

To communicate divers use internationally recognized hand signals. These signals are part of the skills that you must learn when working on your first diving licence. For safe diving it is necessary to perform and interpret the hand signals well. Misunderstanding of them can lead to stress, panic and fatal accidents.

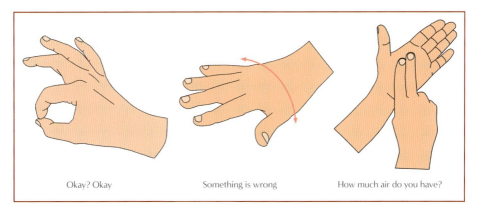

Figure 1.1.5 Some of the internationally recognized diving hand signals. Clear communication above and under the water surface is necessary for safe and enjoyable diving
Copyright by Lars Behnke, apporiented.com

Freediving

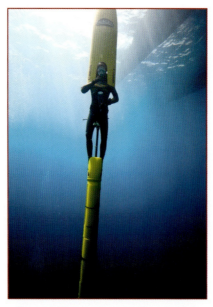

Figure 1.1.6 Freediver Herbert Nitsch
Photo: Francine Kreiss, freediver and underwater photographer

Besides scuba diving, there is another way of diving, which is called *freediving*. Freediving is diving without compressed air but *with one breath*.

The deepest freedive world records at the time of writing:

- A 128-metre world record *constant weight with fins* (swimming under one's own power with fins or a monofin) by the Russian Alexey Molchanov in 2013.[12]

- A 214-metre *no-limits* world record ratified by AIDA (International Association for the Development of Apnea) made by the Austrian Herbert Nitsch in 2007. *No-limits* means 'To dive as deep as possible with an assisted descend with a weight, return with a lifting balloon'.[13]

- The longest *static apnoea dive* world record (holding breath under water without swimming a distance) is 11 minutes and 35 seconds by the Frenchman Stéphane Mifsud (2009).[14]

---

12 Koe, F. (2013) 'Suunto Vertical Blue 2013 Kicks Off This Weekend', Deeper Blue, www.deeperblue.com/suunto-vertical-blue-2013-kicks-weekend (accessed 6 August 2017).

13 Rösken, R., *A Historical Introduction to Breath-Hold Diving and Present-Day Freediving Practice: A Comprehensive Textbook of (Patho)Physiology and Medicine of Apnoea Diving*, N.A.M. Schellart (ed.) Stichting Duik Research, Amsterdam, 2014 (p.9).

14 AIDA – International Association for the Development of Apnea, Symbol of Freediving: World Records, www.aidainternational.org/WorldRecords#recordsMan (accessed 12 September 2017).

EAR, NOSE AND THROAT DISORDERS

Freedivers, also called *apnoea divers* or *breath hold divers*, are dealing in particular with risks regarding the lungs (barotrauma), heart and blood circulation. Freedivers who train for competitions and world records usually want to reach enormous depths and they demand a lot of themselves, searching for their physical limits. As freedivers dive with one breath the problems are partly different to those for scuba divers. Scuba divers dive with compressed air and breathe in and out continuously during the whole dive, which results in a higher level of nitrogen absorbed in the tissues. A scuba dive can take one hour or more depending on the depth of the dive. Freedivers make relatively much shorter dives (a couple of minutes) and the amount of nitrogen in the body is from the breath-taking before going under water and what is stored in the body from previous dives.

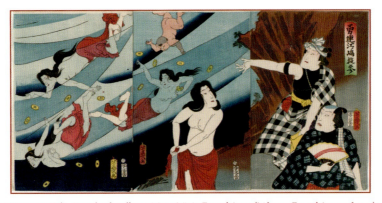

Figure 1.1.7 'A Band of gallant Men Visit Enoshima (Yûren Enoshima yûsan): Actors Ichikawa Kodanji IV and Ichimura Kakitsu IV, with Diving Women'. In this perfectly conserved woodblock print we see female divers collecting golden coins thrown in the water by men. It is likely that these divers are Ama divers, who usually harvest pearls, sponges, molluscs, shells and fish
Print by Utagawa Yoshiiku (1864), copyright MFA, Boston, USA.

BOX 1.1.3 WATER PEOPLE

In human history there have been *water people* for centuries who performed traditional apnoea diving for harvesting (for example pearls, sponges, molluscs, shells and fish). There are still the *Ama divers* in Japan (who go back to the first century BCE!), the *Bajau divers* in Indonesia, Malaysia and the Philippines, the *Moken* in Thailand and Burma and the *Orang Laut* in Riau.[15]

Professor Erica Schagatay from Sweden did research comparing the underwater working times in Japanese Ama divers and the Bajau divers from the Philippines. The Ama divers, mostly women, collect sea molluscs and

---

15 Schagatay, E., Lodin-Sundström, A. and Abrahamsson, E., 'Underwater working times in two groups of traditional apnea divers in Asia: The Ama and the Bajau', *Diving and Hyperbaric Medicine* (2011) 41, 1, 27–30.

the Bajau divers, mainly men, perform spearfishing. The Ama women in this research (average age 60 years) reached depths of between 5 and 12 metres and their dives lasted about 38 seconds and had a surface interval (the time at the water surface between dives) from 38 seconds. The participating Bajau divers (average age 38 years) made dives of 5 to 7 metres with a duration of 28 seconds, and surface intervals from 19 seconds. The Ama woman spend four hours per day under water (50% diving time) and for the Bajau divers 60 per cent underwater working time was registered.[16,17]

According to Schagatay, the Bajau people almost live in the water.[18] Their houses are built on stilts in the water or they nomadize in house-boats. The women deliver their babies in the ocean and the children swim with their eyes open and see as sharply as above the water surface due to very constricted pupils.

It is interesting that the group of Ama divers included a 97-year-old lady (it is exceptional, of course, to dive at this age) and she mentioned that she maybe should retire to be able to enjoy life ashore for a couple of years... Freediving performed this way seems not to be unhealthy if it is still possible at such a high age!

Protocols

The protocols – or rather *treatment options* – I give can also be used for swimmers, snorkelers and surfers with ear, nose and throat disorders. In the treatment options you will notice a pattern of acupuncture points – opening the nose, sinuses, Eustachian tube and ears – recurring repeatedly, simply because these points are so effective.

I offer an extended point selection because, in addition to the points to open the nose and sinuses and to transform Phlegm, for example, I want you to treat the underlying deficiencies or other energetic disharmonies. Without that you will have no or insufficient effect. 'You have to treat the roots of the tree and not just water the leaves a little bit.'[19] Also, you will then have an elaborate choice of points in case the problem is hard to influence. It is advisable to change some points in each treatment to keep the effect strong and reduce adaptation, and to be able to influence the changing patterns of complaints. When I treat my patients the needling retention time is generally 30 minutes.

. . . .

16   Schagatay, E., Lodin-Sundström, A. and Abrahamsson, E., 'Underwater working times in two groups of traditional apnea divers in Asia: The Ama and the Bajau', *Diving and Hyperbaric Medicine* (2011) 41, 1, 27–30.

17   Schatagay, E., 'Human Natural Diving: History and Physiological Aspects', in N.A.M. Schellart (ed.), *A Comprehensive Textbook of (Patho)Physiology and Medicine of Apnoea Diving*, Capita Selecta Duikgeneeskunde, Volume 13, Stichting Duik Research, Amsterdam, 2014.

18   Schatagay, E., Lecture: 'Human natural diving; history and physiological aspects', Stichting Duik Research, Amsterdam, 2014.

19   Braeckman, B., Jing Ming College, Belgium (personal communication).

EAR, NOSE AND THROAT DISORDERS

> **BOX 1.1.4 ENT IN GENERAL AND IN AVIATION**
>
> The ENT treatments in this book are suitable for ENT disorders in general and those occurring in aviation as well. The insights about the interaction between the ambient pressure and air-filled cavities in the body are not only relevant for ENT problems under the water surface. They contribute to more understanding about the ENT functions and the importance of a well-ventilated ENT area in a wider context.

Needles and Needling

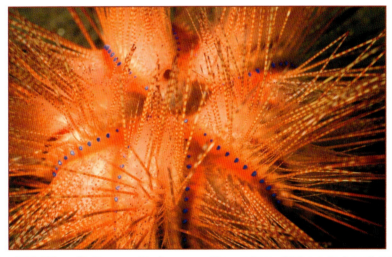

Figure 1.1.8 This radiant sea urchin has many sharp spines which are toxic and painful when you touch them. The spines can break and stick under the skin and cause a severe infection. So you better have acupuncture with sterile disposable needles!
Photo: Janneke Vermeulen, Lembeh Strait, Sulawesi, Indonesia, 2007

The size of needles I use on the body, scalp and face depends on the location and the sensitivity of the patient: 0.25 x 25 mm, 0.25 x 30 mm, 0.25 x 40 mm, 0.16 x 30 mm, 0.18 x 30 mm, 0.20 x 30 mm, 0.20 x 15 mm and 0.16 x 15 mm.

For supplementary ear acupuncture (in addition to acupuncture on the body, scalp and face), a suitable needle size is 0.16–0.17 mm. Semi-permanent auricular needles can also be applied, and retained for a couple of days up to a maximum of one week. I prefer to use Seirin Pyonex press needles (0.22 x 1.6 mm) for sensitive skin and ASP semi-permanent ear needles for normal skin. You also can work with *vaccaria seeds* (small black seeds from the vaccaria plant; apply with medical tape) if someone is too sensitive for semi-permanent needles or when you don't want to penetrate the skin before diving or other watersports.

DIVING MEDICAL ACUPUNCTURE

> **ℹ BOX 1.1.5 SEMI-PERMANENT AURICULAR NEEDLES**
>
> When you treat watersporters with semi-permanent auricular needles they should be removed at least 24 hours before going into the water to prevent a skin infection on the ear. The skin has to be closed totally again before going to dive or swim, else bacteria, viruses or fungi can penetrate the skin.

Acupuncture is *not* just needling some acupuncture points. That's why I want to emphasize that this work also implies putting the right intention on your needles and *be* when you work. Focusing on the Qi and the specific point selection intensifies and determines the effect of your treatment.

Combining acupuncture with supplements, food and lifestyle advice makes your treatment as complete as possible. Chinese herbs can be used as well of course, but I get very good results just with acupuncture, food and lifestyle changes so this book is focused on them.

Clinical Note

When using semi-permanent needles or ear seeds check first that your patient does not have a *plaster allergy* (sensitivity for colophony, also called rosin, which is the yellow sticky substance from pine and spruce tree trunks, used for plaster and tape).

1.2 ANATOMY OF THE EAR
局部解剖

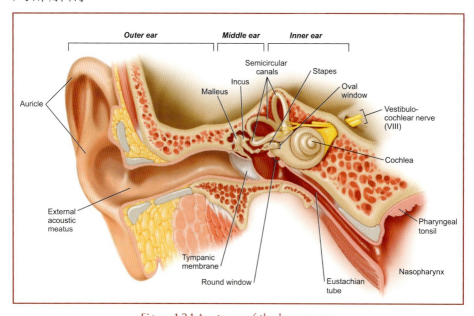

Figure 1.2.1 Anatomy of the human ear

Ear disorders can be divided into:

- external ear disorders
- middle ear disorders
- inner ear disorders.

To understand the pathology of the ear and the most common diving problem, clearing the ears, it's necessary to have some knowledge of the anatomy of the different parts of the ear. In fact the ear is a little world in itself.

- The *external ear* consists of the auricle and the external acoustic meatus (external ear canal).

- The *external* and *middle ear* are separated by the tympanic membrane.

- The *middle ear* consists of the tympanic cavity which contains three tiny bones, the auditory ossicles: the malleus (hammer), incus (anvil) and stapes (stirrup). The middle ear is connected to the Eustachian tube (pharyngotympanic tube). The total length of the Eustachian tube is approximately 36 mm (the cartilaginous part is about 24 mm and the bony part 12 mm).[20]

- The *inner ear* (bony and membranous labyrinth) includes the cochlea and the vestibular organ, and they connect with the vestibulocochlear nerve (balance and hearing nerve). The vestibular organ is divided into three semicircular canals and two otolith organs: the utricle and saccule.

- The three ossicles transmit sounds from the air to the fluid-filled labyrinth. From the labyrinth sound vibrations are transmitted to the brain through the cochlear nerve.

- The Eustachian tube connects the middle ear with the nasopharynx and has the function of regulating the air passage and pressure in the middle ear.

BOX 1.2.1 THE MIDDLE EAR

While diving the *middle ear* is the only air-containing part of the body that needs *active* pressure equalization during the *descent*. So this is obviously the most important area for divers, and has to function well!

An optimally working Eustachian tube is the solution and the first condition for clearing the ears without problems. Swollen mucosa or phlegm

---

20 Singh, V., *Textbook of Anatomy: Head, Neck and Brain*, Volume III, second edition, Reed Elsevier India Private Limited, Haranya, 2014.

in the Eustachian tube can block its free air passage, which is necessary to equalize the pressure in the middle ear and to neutralize the position of the tympanic membrane while descending and ascending.

During the ascent the middle ear usually clears automatically with a properly working Eustachian tube, at a pressure differential of 15 mmHg.[21]

The Valsalva manoeuvre (see Section 1.4) should *not* be used during the ascent as the air-filled cavities expand due to the decrease of the ambient pressure and the diver might risk an overpressure trauma. When clearing the ears is not succeeding during the ascent the diver has to stop ascending. The diver has to descend a little (or can point the affected ear downwards) and then try equalizing again.

1.3 ANATOMY OF THE NOSE AND SINUSES
鼻和鼻窦的解剖

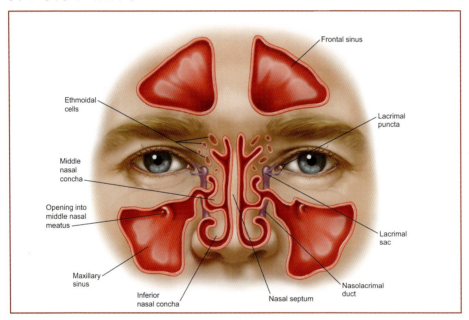

Figure 1.3.1 Anatomy of the nose and sinuses

In addition to the anatomy of the ear it is necessary to have some knowledge of the anatomical structures and functions of the nose and sinuses because they are connected with the middle ear via the Eustachian tube.

---

21 Brandt Corstius, J.J., Dermout, S.M. and Feenstra, L., *Duikgeneeskunde, Theorie en Praktijk*, tweede druk, Elsevier, Amsterdam, 2007.

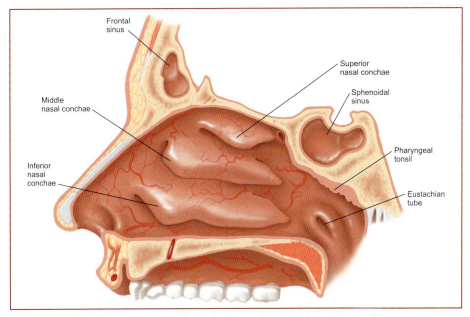

Figure 1.3.2 Side view of the nasal cavity, the frontal and sphenoidal sinuses and the opening of the Eustachian tube

The nose and sinuses comprise:

- nares (nostrils)
- nasal septum
- nasal cavities
- superior, middle and inferior conchae (turbinates)
- superior, middle and inferior meatuses
- nasolacrimal duct
- lacrimal sac
- lacrimal puncta
- frontal sinuses
- ethmoidal sinuses, also called ethmoidal cells
- sphenoidal sinuses
- maxillary sinuses.

The sinuses filter air, produce mucous to moisturize the nasal cavities (divided by the nasal septum), support the resonance of the voice and the sense of smell and, very importantly, they lighten the bones of the skull. The conchae filter, humidify, warm and shape the air we breathe in through the nose. Mucous glands are located in the mucous membranes. Tears, secreted by the lacrimal glands, enter from the corner of the eye through minute openings called puncta to the lacrimal sac, and the nasolacrimal duct brings the fluids to the nasal cavity.

1.4 TECHNIQUES FOR CLEARING THE EARS
清洁中耳道的操作

When you start diving clearing the ears is the first thing you will have to learn. It's a method of equalizing the pressure in the middle ear caused by the ambient pressure. Without clearing the ears diving is not possible. When the Eustachian tube is opened the middle ear can be ventilated and the tympanic membrane can be brought back to its neutral position (this causes a *plopping* sound).

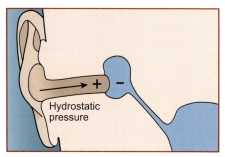

Figure 1.4.1a Underpressure in the middle ear (-) relative to the ambient (hydrostatic) pressure (+) during the descent results in an inward-pulled tympanic membrane

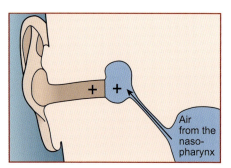

Figure 1.4.1b After equalizing, the tympanic membrane is in neutral position

The Eustachian tube can be blocked due to accumulated phlegm or swollen mucous membranes. In this case it is not possible to get the tympanic membrane back to the middle position (as there is no air flow possible in between the nasopharynx and middle ear). As a result the tension on the membrane will increase. This can lead to very painful sensations in the ear, and descending in the water might be impossible. When the diver ignores the pain during the descent the tension at the tympanic membrane will increase to such an extent that a rupture of the membrane can occur (when there is a differential pressure of 100–150 mmHg[22]). This can be very dangerous. The cold seawater will enter the middle ear and usually cause caloric stimulation of the vestibular organ with violent vertigo and possibly nausea. If the buddy is not alert the diver can lose control, become disoriented and may even drown. The best thing to do in the case of a perforation of the tympanic membrane is to put one finger in the external acoustic meatus so no more seawater can enter the middle ear. This way the temperature in the ear can be regulated and the vertigo will diminish.

It is very important to start clearing the ears immediately when descending through the water. During the first metres the difference in volume is the greatest! The first ten metres you go from 1 ATA at sea level to 2 ATA at ten metres depth. The ambient pressure doubles during that distance. You will have to clear the ears as much as possible and at least once per metre. Three times per metre is often suggested.

Avoiding too rapid and changing vertical displacements is important! Yo-yo actions can trigger ear-clearing problems because the quick changes may irritate the mucous membranes in the Eustachian tube (causing them to swell), especially in the first three metres.

People usually have their first diving lesson in a swimming pool so it is possible to kneel on the bottom of the pool and relax when learning equalizing techniques. Another thing that is taught in that new underwater surroundings is 'Never ascend too quickly!' Climbing too fast can lead to irrevocable damage due to an overpressure injury (e.g. tinnitus due to a rupture of the round or oval window (see Figure 1.2.1, burst lung or decompression illness).

The diver may clear the ears by swallowing (*Toynbee manoeuvre*) or by using the thumb and forefinger of one hand to pinch the nose shut for one to two seconds and trying to breathe out through the nose (*Valsalva manoeuvre*). This brings air to the middle ear and the pressure on the tympanic membrane will neutralize. This technique increases the air pressure in the nasopharynx to 20–100 cmH2O[23] (about 0.02–0.1 ATA) which opens the Eustachian tube.

The Valsalva manoeuvre is fairly safe but if performed too forcefully it can increase the intrathoracic pressure temporarily so that a right–left blood shunt is possible through a *patent foramen ovale* (PFO) in between the right and left atrium in the heart, which can allow nitrogen bubbles to pass into the arterial circulation.[24] These bubbles are able to obstruct arteries and in the worst case this can lead to an arterial gas embolism (AGE) and death. The combination of the Toynbee manoeuvre and the Valsalva manoeuvre is called the *Lowry technique*.

······················

22 Brandt Corstius, J.J., Dermout, S.M. and Feenstra, L., *Duikgeneeskunde, Theorie en Praktijk*, tweede druk, Elsevier, Amsterdam, 2007.
23 Brandt Corstius, J.J., Dermout, S.M. and Feenstra, L., *Duikgeneeskunde, Theorie en Praktijk*, tweede druk, Elsevier, Amsterdam, 2007.
24 One in three people have a PFO, which is a congenital aperture in the septum of the atria. This aperture should close after birth.

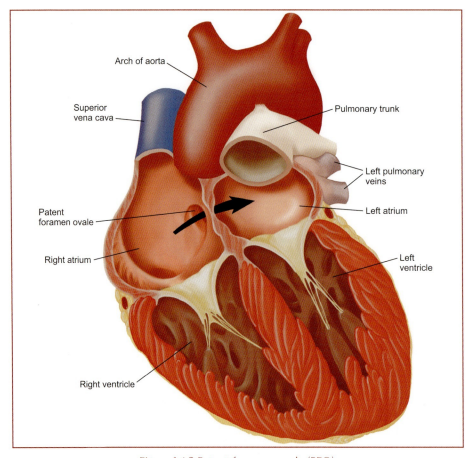

Figure 1.4.2 Patent foramen ovale (PFO)

Another problem besides PFO is when people press too hard with the fingers on the nose while clearing. Capillaries may rupture, and blood in the mask can result in total panic.

Other techniques are:

- The *Edmonds technique*: moving the mandible forward and slightly downward combined with the Toynbee or Valsalva manoeuvre.

- The *Frenzel manoeuvre*: pinching the nose and trying to make a *k sound* (the epiglottis should be closed), bringing the back of the tongue root up, the pharyngeal wall forward and the palate up (this is the beginning of the act of swallowing); like a piston the tongue will push air up.

- The *BTV technique* (Béance tubaire volontaire): a movement like voluntary yawning, which opens the Eustachian tube. This technique is very safe, but can usually only be mastered by very experienced divers.

During the ascent the middle ears usually clear automatically (at a pressure difference of 15 mmHg). Expanding air in the middle ear pushes the Eustachian tube open whereby air flows to the nasopharynx. When ascending one must *not* clear actively by performing the Valsalva manoeuvre because there is a risk of an overpressure barotrauma (equalization by swallowing is safe). An overpressure barotrauma is a trauma caused by differences in pressure while ascending. The ambient pressure decreases during the ascent so the air-filled cavities (e.g. lungs, middle ear) and nitrogen bubbles will expand. Even a small hole in a tooth can result in an explosion of the tooth due to overpressure (so well-kept teeth are important when diving). Breathing out during the ascent and ascending at a certain speed is necessary because that way the lungs can decrease in size, the middle ear can ventilate and nitrogen can leave the body. When clearing the ears is not succeeding during the ascent the diver has to stop ascending. The diver has to descend a little (or can point the affected ear downwards) and then try equalizing again. If equalization is still not possible (due to phlegm or swollen mucous membranes in the Eustachian tube) there is only one solution: to get back to the water surface before running out of air and risking a rupture of the tympanic membrane.

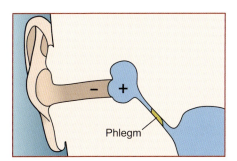

Figure 1.4.3 Phlegm or swollen mucous membranes will block the Eustachian tube, resulting in relative overpressure (+) in the middle ear during the ascent

ⓘ BOX 1.4.1 PROBLEMS WITH EAR CLEARING IN AVIATION

In aviation, aircrew and travellers may also experience equalizing problems. Not being able to clear the ears is the most common medical problem in aviation, as it is in diving.

When the airplane climbs the air pressure in the cabin of the plane is artificially reduced in a relatively short time from 1 ATA to 0.8 ATA. When the plane descends it is returned exactly the other way back to 1 ATA again. An atmosphere of at least 0.8 ATA is needed to supply enough oxygen during the flight. This compares with the air pressure at an altitude of about 2,000 metres (6,561 feet). Outside the airplane, at an altitude of ten kilometres

(32,808 feet) the air pressure is about 0.25 ATA at which the oxygen level is too low to survive.

During the ascent, air in the middle ear expands and the tympanic membrane will be pulled outwards. Normally during the ascent, expanding air in the middle ear pushes the Eustachian tube open automatically (at a pressure difference of 15 mmHg). This allows air to flow to the nasopharynx and the position of the tympanic membrane will be neutralized.

When the plane descends, the air volume in the middle ear decreases and underpressure arises, with an inward-pulled tympanic membrane as a result. During the descent equalization does *not* occur automatically and needs to be done actively.

Ear clearing during the flight can be done by swallowing, chewing, yawning and by performing the Valsalva manoeuvre (in a forceless way!).

Flying with a severe common cold or acute middle ear infection is not recommended because equalization might not be possible, or not sufficiently possible. A squeeze (an underpressure barotrauma) with stabbing pain or even a perforation of the tympanic membrane can be the result.

Sometimes after a flight an ear may be blocked for a couple of hours or weeks accompanied by pain, a feeling of fullness, and deafness. Usually the complaints disappear when the Eustachian tube opens and the air pressure is normalized.

Alternobaric Vertigo

Clearing the ears might cause a typical diving-related dizziness, which is called *alternobaric vertigo*. A difference in pressure in the middle ears might induce dizziness due to a left–right difference in the time it takes for the ears to clear. This occurs in 30 per cent of divers. This dizziness often happens when ascending but it can also be present during descending and after the dive.

According to Brandt Corstius, Dermout and Feenstra (2007), alternobaric vertigo can be prevented most of the time by ascending more slowly, descending a metre or extra swallowing while ascending.[25] The vertigo should pass within 15 minutes – if it does not there might be another problem such as decompression illness, hyperventilation, hypertension or hypotension, hypoglycaemia, a low content of haemoglobin, seasickness or neck problems.

---

25 Brandt Corstius, J.J., Dermout, S.M. and Feenstra, L., *Duikgeneeskunde, Theorie en Praktijk*, tweede druk, Elsevier, Amsterdam, 2007.

⬇ Advice for the Diver and Checks by the Therapist

As an acupuncturist you can give the following advice to the divers in your practice regarding how to clear the ears, such as:

- Take all the time you need to descend in the water.
- Ensure that you stay relaxed.
- Don't rush when other divers descend quickly.
- You and your buddy[26] should agree that the slowest diver sets the pace to prevent ear problems.
- Check while doing the diving medical intake if the diver starts to clear the ears immediately when he or she puts his or her head below the water surface. It's necessary to start clearing the ears directly after bringing the head under the water surface; it is even better to start before the dive if the diver knows he or she experiences equalizing problems quickly/regularly.
- Check if the clearing technique(s) is/are performed well or – if you do not have the skill for that – send the diver to a diving instructor or diving medical physician to check his or her clearing techniques.

Earplugs

Solving the equalization problem by using solid (non-vented) earplugs while diving, which is often suggested by non-diving acupuncturists as an easy solution for this issue, is *not* a good thing. This may lead to eardrum perforation because the plug causes an obstruction in the external acoustic meatus. There will be relative underpressure between the closure (the earplug) and the tympanic membrane when descending because the air between the plug and the tympanic membrane (which has a pressure of 1 ATA at sea level) is compressed, locked up and can't be equalized. Result: overpressure in the middle ear and a pulled outward tympanic membrane. The same thing happens when there is a cerumen plug in the external acoustic meatus.

---

26 One of the diving rules is that you may never dive alone! The diving partner is called a *buddy*.

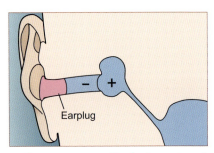

Figure 1.4.4 An earplug or cerumen plug in the external acoustic meatus causes relative underpressure (-) between the plug and the tympanic membrane (during the descent), which results in relative overpressure (+) in the middle ear. The tympanic membrane is pulled outward

Underpressure and Overpressure Injuries

A *squeeze* of the middle ear due to a blocked Eustachian tube or clearing too late is an *underpressure injury*. At the moment there is ear pain, there already has been a squeeze. If the diver ignores pressure and/or pain in the ear while descending (*compression phase*) the tympanic membrane can rupture.

In the case of a middle ear squeeze there is relative underpressure in the middle ear and the tympanic membrane will be pulled inward; small vessels in the tympanic membrane are damaged and there may be a hematoma visible. In addition to pain there might be suction on blood and tissue fluid due to the underpressure. Bleeding thus created gives an increased risk of infection because blood- and tissue fluid-filled cavities are an ideal breeding ground for various forms of bacteria. Bleeding in the middle ear itself can cause a feeling of fullness in the ear. If the tympanic membrane ruptures blood will come out of the ear.

When ascending with a blocked Eustachian tube (this is called a *reverse block*) there might be an *overpressure injury* in the middle ear (the tympanic membrane will be pulled outwards). This can result in pressure, pain, dizziness and tinnitus, and major problems due to the pain getting back to the water surface. When having pain and pressure in the middle ear due to the ascent, these symptoms usually diminish/disappear if you descend a little. During the ascent (decompression phase) you must never perform the Valsalva technique as the air-filled cavities have already expanded due to the diminished ambient pressure!

1.5 DISORDERS THAT MAY CAUSE EQUALIZING PROBLEMS
可能导致平衡障碍的疾患

There are localized physical disorders that can lead to severe problems for divers, such as:

- common cold
- rhinosinusitis

- allergic rhinitis
- hyperreactivity of the mucous membranes in the nose, sinuses and Eustachian tube
- a deviated septum
- a cyst
- a concha bullosa
- a tumour (malignancies are rare in the ENT area and mostly seen in the nasopharynx)
- polyps
- turbinate hypertrophy
- enlarged pharyngeal tonsils (this pathological hypertrophy is also called *adenoids*)[27]
- enlarged lingual tonsils
- enlarged palatine tonsils
- a surplus of cerumen
- ear infections/inflammations.

When experiencing acute problems such as a common cold or allergic rhinitis it is recommended strongly that you do not dive! Clearing the ears and sinuses sufficiently in a safe way is not possible and there is a high risk of barotrauma. Divers sometimes have the tendency to ignore physical signs because they are on a diving holiday for which they have paid a lot of money, which leads to unnecessary problems under water. Even professional divers sometimes ignore pain in their ears because they are focused on the goal of their work.

Regarding ear, nose and throat disorders, I see in my practice mainly divers with *chronic* issues (like allergic rhinitis, hyperreactivity of the mucous membranes, rhinosinusitis) or recurring problems (such as frequently having a common cold) and very occasionally just at the beginning of an acute common cold or at the fourth day when the cold symptoms are still there. Needling on the first day in the case of a common cold can be very effective and result in quick recovery. On the second and third day of an acute cold I don't needle my patients. I advise them to take rest: the virus is still quite infectious and the clinical signs and symptoms usually get worse those days. I instruct them to make ginger or lemon tea with honey depending on whether it is a common cold based on Wind-Cold

---

27 Drake, R.L., Wayne Vogel, A., Mitchell, A.W.M., *Gray's Anatomy for Students*, third edition, Churchill Livingstone Elsevier, Philadelphia, PA, 2015.

or Wind-Heat.[28] It's important that an acute common cold heals well because otherwise there may be secondary infections resulting in rhinosinusitis and ear inflammations.

I experience a lot of Slippery pulses resulting from chronic and/or recurrent ENT issues. A Slippery pulse (*Hua Mai*) is an indication of Dampness and its resultant Phlegm.

Divers who suffer from a common cold, rhinosinusitis, an allergic rhinitis or hyperreactivity of the nasal mucosa can be treated very well by acupuncture, but of course not when the diver is at a diving spot. Lots of divers I see have chronic nasal congestion and discharge based on weak Wei Qi (Defensive Qi), stress, smoking and consuming lots of sugar and/or milk.

It's safer to diving when you treat the complaints and eliminate them totally some time before the diver wants to go diving. It's necessary to improve the energy level and condition of the diver so he or she feels mentally and physically well in addition to having a solid open air passage in the nose, sinuses, Eustachian tube and middle ear.

It's very supportive to give one or two additional treatments just before the holiday to improve the diver's general condition and optimize the ventilation in the Eustachian tube. In the Netherlands some divers test their ears in a swimming pool or lake when they have had a couple of treatments to examine if clearing the ears is going well again before they leave for the holiday. In principle, when you can clear the ears above the water they will be fine under water as long as the diving techniques are performed well.

For chronic ear, nose and throat disorders it is recommended to visit an ENT doctor first to exclude anatomic variations such as nasal septum deviation and concha bullosa. When these factors are causing an obstruction, acupuncture will not be the solution, but they may be an indication for surgery.

Localized and General Causes of Ear-Clearing Problems
Deviated Septum
A deviated septum can cause a blocked nose (at one or both sides) but in that case the only solution is a manual reposition or surgery by an ENT doctor. When a deviation is the result of an external trauma it may be repositioned manually by an ENT doctor in the first days directly after the accident. If the

---

28   The best honey comes directly from a biological beekeeper as the honey is not heated (the nutritional value can be reduced by the heating process) and no sugar water is given to the bees to keep them alive in wintertime. A good medicinal honey is Manuka honey, made from the flower of the Manuka tree (also called the New Zealand tea tree or Leptospermum scoparium) and famous for its antibacterial and antiviral effects. One teaspoon per day is sufficient. A possible side-effect of eating honey is an allergic reaction in people who are allergic to bees. Eating honey from your local area regularly may be very helpful in reducing allergic reactions in general.

obliquity exists for longer than six weeks and causes functional problems surgery is requisite.

Fifty per cent of people with a deviated septum have complaints above the water surface as well. At sea level nasal blockage due to the septum deviation can lead to problems like snoring or dyspnoea. Sleeping on a specific side might not feel good because one side of the nose is blocked due to the deviation. In an airplane clearing the ears might not be possible. When the deviated septum is corrected by surgery a diver needs to wait for two months before starting to dive again. Before this time, simply putting on the mask will be painful. The inside of the nose needs to be healed: there can still be swelling of the mucous membranes, directly after surgery there can be a risk of bleeding, and for the first three weeks blowing the nose is not allowed.

Cyst

A cyst in the maxillary sinus can block the central duct but often a maxillary sinus cyst is asymptomatic and incidentally found on an X-ray. If it causes problems, surgery is needed.

Concha Bullosa

A concha bullosa is an air-filled cavity, mostly seen in the middle concha. This pneumatization occurs as a result of migration of ethmoidal cells to the concha. A concha bullosa can block the maxillary sinus, in which case the lateral aspect needs to be removed.

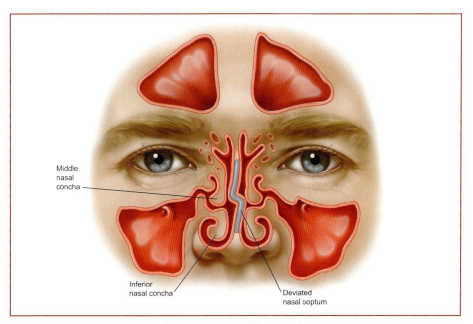

Figure 1.5.1 Deviation of the nasal septum

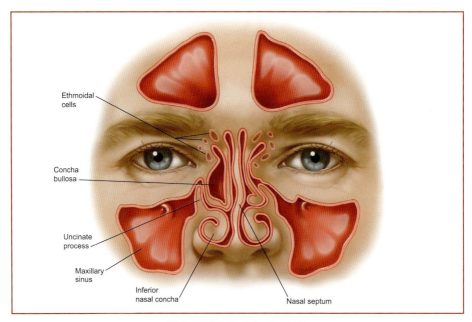

Figure 1.5.2 Concha bullosa

Polyps

Polyps are benign lesions on the mucosa in the nasal cavity and sinuses. They can block the nasal and sinus passages in which case equalization is not possible. In severe cases surgery might be needed.

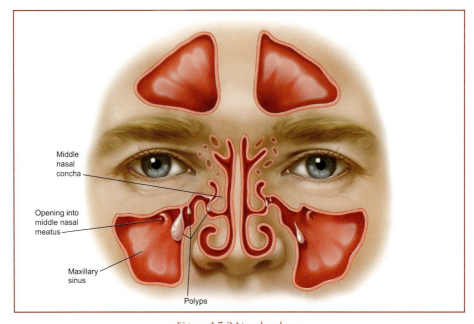

Figure 1.5.3 Nasal polyps

Cerumen

The presence of a cerumen plug in the ear, which is natural ear discharge (*earwax*), can lead to a blockage of the external acoustic meatus when descending in the water. Cerumen swells in water whereby it can block the ear canal, resulting in an external ear squeeze. In this case there is air (with a pressure of 1 ATA from sea level) locked up between the cerumen plug and the tympanic membrane. When descending the air will be compressed due to the increasing ambient pressure resulting in a vacuum (relative underpressure) in the space between the cerumen plug and tympanic membrane (as no equalization of this part is possible). This vacuum results in relative overpressure in the middle ear and the tympanic membrane is pulled outward. The tympanic membrane can perforate if the pressure and/or pain are ignored in case the diver descends further into the water. When performing the Valsalva maneuver in this situation there is even more risk of a perforation of the tympanic membrane. A *cap that is too tight* and a *non-vented earplug* can block the external acoustic meatus in the same way. When the cap is too tight the diver can simply make a small hole on both sides of the cap so the water can enter the cap and the external acoustic meatus and neutralize the vacuum situation.

Note: Cerumen creates an acidic coating in the external acoustic meatus and is water repellent. Using ear swabs regularly can damage the hair cells that remove the cerumen and can irritate the cerumen-producing glands and activate them too much.

Yo-Yo Actions

Yo-yo actions are mostly experienced by divers with less experience and thus insufficient buoyancy techniques. They go up and down instead of being able to stay at one level. These yo-yo actions can irritate the mucous membranes (causing them to swell), especially in the first three metres. Yo-yo actions also may occur when diving instructors have to go up and down a lot to help students during their first diving lessons.

Smoking

Nicotine irritates the mucous membranes and leads to the production of mucus, which can block the nose, the Eustachian tube and/or the sinuses.

Premenstrual Oedema

Due to fluctuations in oestrogen and progesterone an excess of aldosterone may occur. This increase can cause fluid retention in the mucous membranes, which might lead to congestion in the Eustachian tube. Acupuncture can help balance the hormonal system (add combination **KI-27** Shufu and **KI-6** Zhaohai) to reduce the retention of fluids (Jin Ye; see Box 1.7.5).

Pharyngeal, Palatine and Lingual Tonsils

Enlarged pharyngeal, palatine and/or lingual tonsils, which still can occur in adulthood, can block the nose, Eustachian tube and/or throat and make clearing the ears impossible. In general a blocked Eustachian tube due to an enlarged pharyngeal tonsil might decrease hearing and induce middle ear infections. Swollen palatine and/or lingual tonsils impede trouble-free swallowing. If there is tonsillitis (caused by a bacterium or virus) you can treat it in an appropriate manner so the tonsils can shrink again. Surgery is an option to treat this condition if it becomes chronic.

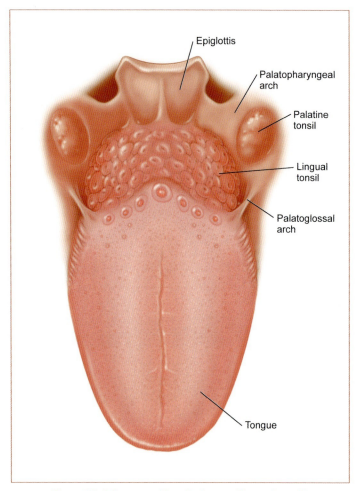

Figure 1.5.4 Tongue with palatine and lingual tonsils

Clearing Techniques

Poorly performed techniques can lead to problems with clearing the ears. Good education at a qualified diving school is important to learn diving in a safe and proper way. The diver has to start clearing the ears immediately when descending (in the first metre). To prevent problems it is best to start clearing the moment the face and nose contact the water and the hair is still above the water surface. To clear the ears correctly it is important to keep the head in a higher position than the feet when descending.

Stress

Stress can be expressed by clamping on the regulator. Clamping can give contractions in the tensor veli palatini muscle, which opens the Eustachian tube; but when not working well it will not effectively open the Eustachian tube (see Figure 2.6b), resulting in possible equalization difficulties.

Ciliary System

The *ciliary system* extending from the nose to the middle ear is sensitive to:

- temperature changes (cold ➔ warm, warm ➔ cold)
- humidity
- smoking
- alcohol
- medication
- disturbed day/night system
- repeated dives
- tiredness
- air conditioning (plane, diving accommodation, hotel).

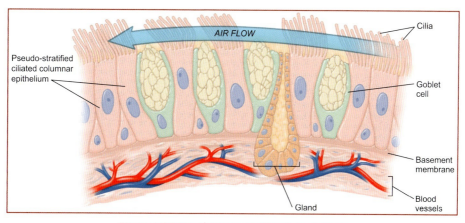

Figure 1.5.5 Nasal mucosa with ciliary system

Diving can irritate the mucous membranes because:

- the compressed air in the tank is dry and cold

- in tropical zones the surface water is often warm and deeper in the water it's usually colder; there can also be currents of water with different temperatures (the mucous membranes can react to these temperature changes)

- the sea water is salty and there are a lot of microbes living in the ocean (for example, the corals are full of microbes); before you put on your mask the sea water can enter the nose and irritate/infect the mucosa.

- of yo-yo actions.

The nose is essential for divers, in the first place to be able to smell if the compressed air in the tank is clean when preparing the equipment before diving. Clean air has no smell. Breathing in contaminated air can be very dangerous for the health of the diver. Symptoms caused by breathing in bad gas (e.g. rust, contaminants produced by a compressor, too much carbon monoxide or carbon dioxide) are headache, nausea, tiredness or vision problems. In the worst case impure air may lead to unconsciousness under water.

Diving Medical Intake

When a diver comes for an acupuncture treatment it's important to check diving-related aspects besides doing the regular medical history. Recreational divers are strongly recommended to use a logbook (when you arrive at a diving resort, you can show this to give details of your most recent dive). You normally get a logbook from the diving organization when you accomplish your first diving license. Professional divers may be legally obliged to maintain a logbook. The logbook will give details of dives made including depth of diving, diving time, name of your buddy, details of the dive itself (shark, turtle) and a signature of the instructor/Divemaster (when the diving is organized by a diving school/diving resort/live-a-board).

A logbook contributes to safety, as it can include diving medical information like diving medical examinations.

Check the following data when you conduct the intake:

- Which certification does the diver have?

- How many dives has the diver made?

- What is the frequency of diving?

- When did the problems start (i.e. which dive/date/period)?

- At which moment or which depth do the problems start?
- Do the problems maintain under water or not?
- What is the diver doing when the problems occur? Ignoring them? Stopping the dive?
- Has the way of clearing the ears been checked by a professional like a Divemaster, an instructor or diving medicine doctor?
- Did the diver visit a doctor before coming for acupuncture?
- Is there a drugs prescription?
- Is the diver smoking or using alcohol?
- Has the diver been examined to be fit for diving or not?
- Is there a diving holiday scheduled or is the diver following a course to upgrade his or her diving techniques?

Here is a schedule from the RSTC[29] diving licences to get an idea what kind of licences there are:

- Open Water Diver (maximum depth of 18 metres)
- Advanced Diver (maximum depth of 30 metres)
- Rescue Diver
- Divemaster (you need 60 logged dives when you want to start your Divemaster course)
- Instructor.

1.6 COMMON COLD
感冒
Western Medicine
Definition and Aetiology

The common cold or nasopharyngitis is an acute viral infection in the upper respiratory tract. There are more than 200 types of viruses that can cause a common cold. Frequently seen viruses are rhinovirus, coranovirus, adenovirus, parainfluenza virus and the human respiratory syncytial virus. Viruses enter our system by the nose or mouth. When there is a sudden difference in external temperature of more than 7 degrees Celsius the cilia in the nose collapse and a virus can penetrate the body.

---

29 RSTC stands for Recreational Scuba Training Council, and includes the organizations PADI, DAN, SDI, SSI, PDA, IDEA, PDIC, ACUC, IAC, IDA, IDDA, NASDS, PSS and VIT.

The common cold is the most seen infectious disease, with possible secondary complications in the sinuses, ears, throat and lungs. It involves absenteeism from work and school, reduced productivity and high medical costs. This implies that knowledge about the common cold and its prevention (e.g. by regular hand washing to remove viruses) is not only important regarding equalizing problems experienced by divers but with respect to an optimal general health.

In Chinese medicine there are opportunities to prevent a common cold. The common cold is related to Wei Qi, emotional functioning, the general energy level and the immune system of the person. The stronger the Wei Qi and the immune system are, the less chance there is a person gets a common cold.

What I see in my practice is that people who have had acupuncture in the past to improve their immune system do not get a common cold or flu as often as they did in the past. For example, they don't get ill when their family members have a common cold whereas in the past they would always get sick at the same time. Maybe this is not evidence-based practice but my Dutch patients are very grounded and not willing to pay for a treatment when it's not effective.

One of the standard points I use in almost all my ENT treatments is **LU-7** Lieque, because it fortifies Lung-Qi and harmonizes the emotions (especially releasing sadness, grief and worries). In particular chronic stress supresses the immune system, which raises the risk of a viral infection like the common cold. This implies that emotional balance is essential in maintenance of the immune system. This is why **SP-6** Sanyinjiao is also a favourite point. According to Aung and Chen (2007)[30] it has as indications 'general tonification, immune enhancement', which is of great importance in cases of recurring or chronic ENT pathology. **ST-36** Zusanli tonifies the Qi of the whole body and supports the immune system by 'inhibiting inflammatory reactions'.[31]

Treatment

The Western treatment of a common cold is basically focused on reducing the swelling of the mucous membranes. It is recommended strongly not to dive when having a common cold as there is a big risk of barotrauma of the middle ears and sinuses!

Otrivin® nose drops: Otrivin® (xylometazoline) is very effective for a common cold in reducing the congestion in the nasal cavities and Eustachian tube. Regarding the occurrence of equalizing problems in general, Otrivin® might be applied as a *preventive* with diving, although opinions vary, according to Brandt Corstius,

---

30   Aung, S.K.H. and Chen, W.P.D., *Clinical Introduction to Medical Acupuncture*, Thieme, New York, 2007 (p.38).
31   Xia, Y., Ding, G. and Wu, G.-C., *Current Research in Acupuncture*, Springer Science+Business Media, New York, 2013 (p.284).

Dermout and Feenstra (2007).[32] A side-effect of Otrivin® is a rebound effect and this is especially dangerous when making several dives per day. When the mucous membranes start to swell at the moment the diver wants to ascend a reverse block might occur.

Using Otrivin® as a preventive before one dive per day during a one-week diving holiday is no problem and in that case it is best applied just before the dive.

People who use Otrivin® daily can become addicted to it and maintain a problem due to the rebound effect. Acupuncture can be very helpful for breaking through this addiction by decreasing the swelling of the mucous membranes and support their blood circulation. Usually three to four acupuncture sessions will be enough to stop the daily need for Otrivin® but some more treatments might be needed for a long-term open air passage.

As mentioned above, using Otrivin® occasionally, such as once a day during a one-week diving holiday or when used just once during a flight for a vacation or business trip, is not a problem, but using it for longer than seven days can impair the mucous membranes.

Not needing xylometazoline at all would be best, of course. Salty nose drops are a better solution for the long term as they moisten the dehydrated mucous membranes (e.g. for flight staff, or office people in climate-controlled buildings where dry air is a continuous factor).

Sudafed® tablets: Sudafed® (pseudoephedrine) is a decongestant and is used as preventive for equalizing problems with diving. It's effective when there is a light squeeze of the middle ear.[33] Sudafed® gives no rebound effect at the mucosa but can cause cardiac arrhythmia and high blood pressure. Sudafed® is not sold in the Netherlands but is available in the USA.

Painkillers: Paracetamol or NSAIDs (non-steroidal anti-inflammatory drugs like ibuprofen and naproxen) are used to treat pain and fever. Codeine (an opioid) has a cough-suppressing effect and might be prescribed in the case of a persisting tickling cough (though not in the first two days of a common cold as mucus should be discharged). Codeine has sedative side-effects and should not be used before diving as it can provoke nitrogen narcosis; also, diving with a cough is discouraged strongly.

Vitamin C is advised to support the general condition, especially in the case of physical stress.

---

32 Brandt Corstius, J.J., Dermout, S.M. and Feenstra, L., *Duikgeneeskunde, Theorie en Praktijk*, tweede druk, Elsevier, Amsterdam, 2007.
33 Brandt Corstius, J.J., Dermout, S.M. and Feenstra, L., *Duikgeneeskunde, Theorie en Praktijk*, tweede druk, Elsevier, Amsterdam, 2007.

Clinical Notes

Nitrogen narcosis is a narcotic state of the brain caused by increased partial pressure of nitrogen (partial pressure is the pressure of a specific gas in a mix of gases), with possible signs and symptoms like drowsiness, loss of reality, euphoria and irrational acts. It is also called *depth drunkenness*. Usually nitrogen narcosis can be felt at depths of 30 metres and over but is dependent on the person's sensitivity to it. When nitrogen narcosis occurs the diver should ascend to shallower water until the signs and symptoms resolve.

Chinese Medicine
Definition and Aetiology

The common cold belongs to the Shang Feng Gan Mao disorders, which means *Injuries by Wind*. Wind accompanied by exogenous pathogenic factors (Cold, Heat, Dampness, Dryness) enters the body. Wind penetrates through the skin pores, the nose and mouth. This can happen when the Wei Qi is not strong enough to protect the body, which can be in general or temporarily, or when the pathogenic factor is very strong and able to pass through the surface of the body.

Sudden changes in weather/climate and moving from climate-controlled surroundings to outdoors can be triggers for 'catching wind', as they say literally in China.[34,35]

Besides protecting the body, the Wei Qi warms the surface of the body and regulates the body temperature by opening and closing the pores. The Wei Qi circulates on the surface of the body, in the space between the skin and muscles. Weak Wei Qi can result in frequent common cold and in difficulty regulating body temperature.

The Wei Qi circulates 25 times in the day in the exterior (Yang level) and 25 times in the night in the interior (Yin level).

During sleep Wei Qi goes into the interior of the body and the exterior of the body is unprotected. When the surface of the body is not protected by an external covering, Wind can gain access to the body more easily. This can be seen, for example, when sleeping next to an open window, in climate-control environments or when no blanket is used.[36]

Sleeping in an airplane with cold and dry climate-control during a long-distance flight with insufficient body protection can contribute to developing

---

34 Maclean, W. and Lyttleton, J., *Clinical Handbook of Internal Medicine*, Volume 1, fifth printing, University of Western Sydney, Sydney, 2008.
35 Xie, Z.F. and Liao, J.Z., *Traditional Chinese Medicine*, Foreign Languages Press, Beijing, 1993.
36 Maclean, W. and Lyttleton, J., *Clinical Handbook of Internal Medicine*, Volume 1, fifth printing, University of Western Sydney, Sydney, 2008.

a common cold just before arriving at the diving destination and ruining the holiday.

Some people already sit in the plane wearing summer clothes because they are going to a tropical destination not realizing that the plane might be very cold and just a blanket might not be sufficient during travel time. Diving holidays need to be prepared for very carefully as divers usually take their own diving equipment and/or underwater cameras. They should prioritize taking care of their health as well, but often they do not consider easy solutions that can protect them during the flight such as a shawl or a fleece jacket with a hood.

Deadman, Al-Khafaji and Baker (2015) describe the origin of Wei Qi clearly, as follows:

> Defensive qi is considered to be a part of the original qi which has its origin in the Kidney's pre heaven qi (lower jiao). It is constantly nourished by the post-heaven essence of water and grain produced by the action of the Stomach and Spleen on food (middle jiao). Finally, it is the Lung which controls the defensive qi and spreads it to the surface of the whole body (upper jiao). It is therefore said that the root of the defensive qi is in the lower jiao, it is nourished by the middle jiao and it spreads in the upper jiao, and this is clarified by the observation that a person's defensive qi may be insufficient due to congenital weakness, inadequate diet or upper jiao deficiency.[37]

Clinical Signs and Symptoms of a Common Cold

- Nasal congestion or rhinorrhoea (discharge)
- Sneezing
- Sore throat
- Cough
- Lacrimation
- Aversion to cold
- Headache
- Fever
- Chills
- Body aches.

---

37 Deadman, P., Al-Khafaji, M. and Baker, K., *A Manual of Acupuncture*, Journal of Chinese Medicine Publications, Hove, 2015 (p.347).

Normally it takes three to seven days to recover from a common cold. When mismanaged or not resolved it can take up to several weeks.

In the section 'Pattern Differentiation' below I have subdivided the most frequently seen patterns, of which Wind-Cold, Wind-Heat and Summer-Heat with Dampness are the most common ones. The main treatment principles and selection of the acupuncture points are related to the common cold type and the presenting pulse and tongue diagnosis. I will mention the most important points to influence the specific condition and the corresponding clinical signs and symptoms – from which you can choose the needed selection for your patient – and points to support general tonification and the immune system. When people have recurring common colds it is necessary to treat the underlying deficiency, and in the case of an acute common cold the person will feel much better when you support general tonification and immunity besides treating the present clinical signs and symptoms.

Pattern Differentiation
1 Wind-Cold
An invasion of Wind-Cold enters through the skin pores, constricts the Wei Qi, attacks primarily the Bladder and Small Intestine channels and blocks the descending and diffusing of Lung-Qi (thereby causing Jin Ye to stagnate and accumulate, congealing into Phlegm).

> **BOX 1.6.1 COMMON COLD: WIND-COLD ATTACK**
>
> Wind-Cold → Constricts Wei Qi → Circulation ↓
> (no sweating, cold shivers, body aches)
>
> → Blocks Lung → Descending and diffusing of Qi ↓
> (sneezing, wheezing, cough)
>
> → Descending and diffusing of Jin Ye ↓
> (nasal discharge, sputum)

● Clinical Signs and Symptoms
- Nasal congestion or thin watery or white discharge
- Cough and coughing up thin watery sputum
- Wheezing
- Sneezing
- Lacrimation

- No fever or mild fever and predominantly chills
- No sweating (the pores are closed by the cold)
- Occipital headache and stiff neck
- Body aches
- Aversion to cold
- Pale urine.

Pulse: Floating (*Fu*) and Tight (*Jin*).

Tongue: Normal (in the initial stage) or with a thin and white coating.

Season: Wind-Cold mainly occurs in autumn and winter (and may be caused by climate-control).

● Treatment Principle
- Expel Wind-Cold.
- Promote the descending and diffusing of Lung-Qi.
- Open the nose.

● Acupuncture Points (select from)

LI-4 Hegu, **LU-7** Lieque, **TB-5** Waiguan, **BL-12** Fengmen, **BL-13** Feishu, **LI-20** Yingxiang, **M-HN-3** Yintang, **GB-20** Fengchi, **SP-6** Sanyinjiao, **ST-36** Zusanli, **CV-6** Qihai.

● Explanation
- **LI-4**, **LU-7** and **TB-5** expel Wind-Cold and release the exterior. **LI-4** adjusts sweating (opens the pores) and regulates Wei Qi.
- **LU-7**, **BL-12** and **BL-13** promote the descending and diffusing of Lung-Qi (cough). Use **BL-12** in the early stage of the condition and **BL-13** in the case of recurring pathology.
- **LI-20** and Yintang expel Wind and open the nose (congestion, discharge, sneezing).
- **GB-20** eliminates Wind from the head. Add in the case of blocked ears, a stiff neck, headache or lacrimation.
- **SP-6** and **ST-36** support general tonification and immunity.

- **CV-6** fortifies Qi in general (low energy level in the case of recurrent and chronic ENT pathology).

- Moxa to eliminate the Cold: **GB-20**, **TB-5** and **ST-36**.

● Clinical Notes

- Besides regulating, **LI-4** might tonify Wei Qi[38] in combination with **ST-36** and **CV-6** Qihai.[39] This action is important regarding the prevention of ENT disorders caused by Wind. A tonifying needle technique should be performed when the acute clinical signs and symptoms are no longer present.

- **TB-5** can be used 'for all wind, cold, summer-heat and damp pathogens, headaches and fever'[40] and is especially effective at the start of a common cold.

- **BL-12** is useful for early stages of all Wind conditions to release the exterior, and strengthens Wei Qi. According Soulié de Morant[41] this point works as a preventive against flu and diseases caused by Cold.

- **BL-13** is a key point (Back Shu Point) for all Lung disorders (especially chronic pathology where tonification of Lung-Qi or Lung-Yin is needed). Add this point combined with **BL-12** for recurring common colds.

- **SP-6** is important in recurrent and chronic ENT disorders combined with disturbed emotions (in particular overthinking).

● Food

Fresh ginger tea with honey. Take one and a half litres of water and a piece of ginger (5–6 cm). Peel the ginger and cut it into small pieces. Boil the water with the ginger pieces for about ten minutes. Finish by adding two tablespoons of honey when the ginger tea is ready.[42]

Ginger is pungent and induces sweating. When the pores open the Wind-Cold pathogen can be expelled. Ginger transforms Phlegm and relieves a cough.

According to a study by Chang *et al.* (2013), fresh, but not dried, ginger (Zingiber officinale) has anti-viral activity against human respiratory syncytial

---

38 Maciocia, G., *De Grondslagen van de Chinese Geneeskunde, Een Complete Basishandleiding voor Acupuncturisten en Fytotherapeuten, Tweede Uitgave*, Churchill Livingstone, New York, 2005.
39 Deadman, P., Al-Khafaji, M. and Baker, K., *A Manual of Acupuncture*, Journal of Chinese Medicine Publications, Hove, 2015.
40 Deadman, P., Al-Khafaji, M. and Baker, K., *A Manual of Acupuncture*, Journal of Chinese Medicine Publications, Hove, 2015 (pp.396, 397).
41 Boermeester, W., *Tekstboek Acupunctuur, deel I, Punten*, Chinese Medicine Data, Kapellen, 1989.
42 Bridges, L.P., The Hague, the Netherlands, 2011 (personal communication).

virus (HRSV) in both upper and lower human respiratory tract cell lines.[43] This research concretizes that fresh ginger is medically effective by blocking the viral attachment and internalization of HRSV-induced plaque formation on airway epithelium.[44] Besides its anti-viral activity against HRSV, ginger has an 'anti-rhinoviral effect',[45] which makes ginger useful (in particular as a preventive) against viral airway infections (besides that, ginger has 'anti-microbial activities against various bacteria, fungi and nematodes'[46]).

2 Wind-Heat

An invasion of Wind-Heat enters via the nose and mouth. The descending and diffusing of Lung-Qi is obstructed, while Heat dries and damages Jin Ye.

There is a slight aversion to cold as Wind-Heat obstructs Wei Qi, whereby the muscles cannot be warmed[47] (so it is important to cover the body).

● Clinical Signs and Symptoms

- Nasal congestion or thick yellow or green discharge
- Sore throat
- High fever and mild chills or no chills
- Cough and coughing up thick yellow sputum
- Sneezing
- Sweating
- Frontal headache, or a headache in the whole head
- Slight aversion to cold
- Scanty dark urine
- Thirst.

---

43 Chang, J.S., Wang, K.C., Yeh, C.F., Shieh, D.E. and Chiang, L.C., 'Fresh ginger (Zingiber officinale) has anti-viral activity against human respiratory syncytial virus in human respiratory tract cell line', *Journal of Ethnopharmacology* (2013) 145, 1, 146–151.

44 Chang, J.S., Wang, K.C., Yeh, C.F., Shieh, D.E. and Chiang, L.C., 'Fresh ginger (Zingiber officinale) has anti-viral activity against human respiratory syncytial virus in human respiratory tract cell line', *Journal of Ethnopharmacology* (2013) 145, 1, 146–151.

45 Denyer *et al.* (1994) quoted by Chang, J.S., Wang, K.C., Yeh, C.F., Shieh, D.E. and Chiang, L.C., 'Fresh ginger (Zingiber officinale) has anti-viral activity against human respiratory syncytial virus in human respiratory tract cell line', *Journal of Ethnopharmacology* (2013) 145, 1, 146–151 (p.149).

46 Ali *et al.* 2008 quoted by Chang, J.S., Wang, K.C., Yeh, C.F., Shieh, D.E. and Chiang, L.C., 'Fresh ginger (Zingiber officinale) has anti-viral activity against human respiratory syncytial virus in human respiratory tract cell line', *Journal of Ethnopharmacology* (2013) 145, 1, 146–151 (p.147).

47 Maciocia, G., *The Practice of Chinese Medicine: The Treatment of Diseases with Acupuncture and Chinese Herbs*, Churchill Livingstone, Edinburgh, 1994.

Pulse: Floating (*Fu*) and Rapid (*Shuo*).

Tongue: Normal (in the initial stage) or red front with a thin and slight yellow coating.

Season: Wind-Heat presents mostly in spring and summer.

● Treatment Principle

- Expel Wind-Heat.
- Clear Heat from the Lung.
- Promote the descending and diffusing of Lung-Qi.
- Open the nose.

● Acupuncture Points (select from)

LI-4 Hegu, **LI-11** Quchi, **TB-5** Waiguan, **LU-5** Chize, **LU-10** Yuji, **LU-11** Shaoshang, **LU-7** Lieque, **BL-12** Fengmen, **BL-13** Feishu, **LI-20** Yingxiang, **M-HN-3** Yintang, **GB-20** Fengchi, **GV-14** Dazhui, **ST-44** Neiting, **SP-6** Sanyinjiao, **ST-36** Zusanli.

● Explanation

- **LI-4**, **LI-11** and **TB-5** expel Wind-Heat and release the exterior.
- **LU-5** (cough) and **LU-10** (no voice) clear Heat from the Lung.
- **LU-11** expels Wind-Heat (sore throat).
- **LU-7**, **BL-12** and **BL-13** promote the descending and diffusing of Lung-Qi. Use **BL-12** in the early stage of the condition and **BL-13** in recurring pathology.
- **LI-20** and Yintang expel Wind-Heat and open the nose.
- **GB-20** eliminates Wind from the head. Add if there is a headache.
- **GV-14** and **ST-44** clear Heat. Use when there is fever. **ST-44** also helps for pain and swelling of the throat.
- **SP-6** and **ST-36** support general tonification and immunity.

● Clinical Notes

- According to Aung and Chen (2007) **LI-11** has as one of its indications 'immune enhancing'.[48] Important for recurring common colds.

---

48 Aung, S.K.H. and Chen, W.P.D., *Clinical Introduction to Medical Acupuncture*, Thieme, New York, 2007 (p.28).

- **LU-10** is very effective when having *no voice*. After needling the voice can return in one day. You can instruct your patient to perform acupressure on **LU-10**, both sides, to support the treatment.

- In the case of an extreme sore throat/laryngitis you can perform a blood-letting technique on **LU-11** to reduce Heat.

● Food

Take the juice of half a lemon in a mug with hot water and add some honey. In Chinese medicine lemon has a sour (astringent) flavour and cooling property and generates Yin Fluids (Xue (Blood), Jin Ye (Body Fluids) and Jing (Essence)). Seen with Western eyes, lemon is high in antioxidants and vitamin C and alkalizes the body. Lemon (Citrus lemon L.) peel has 'antimicrobial activity'.[49] 'Citrus flavonoids have a large spectrum of biological activity including antibacterial, antifungal, antidiabetic, anticancer and antiviral activities (Burt 2004; Ortuno *et al.* 2006)' (Dhanavade *et al.* 2011).[50]

Honey is neutral and sweet (neutralizes the sourness of lemon), moistens the throat and relieves a cough.

3 Summer-Heat with Dampness

Summer-Heat with Dampness or Summer-Humidness can occur in humid hot surroundings where usually lots of beautiful diving places are located, like the Philippines, the Maldives and Micronesia. Wind is the pathogenic factor that invades the body and carries Summer-Heat-Dampness. Summer-Humidness often happens in late summer/early autumn, for example when wearing wet clothes for too long after heavy rain or when returning by boat after diving (sitting in wet swimwear on a very windy deck on a boat). Tropical rains can be short but very intense, especially in the wet monsoon season. Dampness is heavy, turbid and sticky and invades the Spleen and Stomach in particular.

● Clinical Signs and Symptoms

- A feeling of cloth wrapped around the head, foggy head, not clear thinking

- General heaviness of the body and body aches

- Digestive problems like nausea, vomiting, poor appetite and loose stools

---

[49] Dhanavade, M.J., Jalkute, C.B., Sonawane, K.D and Ghosh, J., 'Study antimicrobial activity of lemon (*Citrus lemon* L.) peel extract, *British Journal of Pharmacology and Toxicology (2010)* 2, 3, 119–122.

[50] Dhanavade, M.J., Jalkute, C.B., Sonawane, K.D and Ghosh, J., 'Study antimicrobial activity of lemon (*Citrus lemon* L.) peel extract, *British Journal of Pharmacology and Toxicology (2010)* 2, 3, 119–122 (p.119).

- Feeling worse in the mid-afternoon[51]
- Nasal congestion or white and sticky discharge
- Slight sweating
- Relatively high fever, aversion to cold
- Mild cough
- Sore throat
- White or yellow sticky sputum
- Tiredness
- Irritability and restlessness
- Yellow and scanty urine.

Pulse: Soggy (*Ru*) and Rapid (*Shuo*).

Tongue: Thick and sticky white or yellow coating.

Season: Summer-Heat with Dampness occurs often in late summer and early autumn (and in tropical/subtropical regions).

● Treatment Principle

— Expel Wind-Damp-Heat.

— Promote the descending and diffusing of Lung-Qi.

— Resolve Dampness.

— Open the nose.

● Acupuncture Points (select from)
LI-4 Hegu, **LI-11** Quchi, **TB-5** Waiguan, **LU-7** Lieque, **SP-9** Yinlingquan, **CV-12** Zhongwan, **LU-10** Yuji, **LU-11** Shaoshang, **LI-20** Yingxiang, **M-HN-3** Yintang, **ST-25** Tianshu, **PC-6** Neiguan, **SP-6** Sanyinjiao, **ST-36** Zusanli.

● Explanation

- **LI-4**, **LI-11** and **TB-5** expel Wind-Heat and release the exterior. **TB-5** treats external Damp pathogens as well.
- **LU-7** promotes the descending and diffusing of Lung-Qi (cough).

---

[51] Maclean, W. and Lyttleton J., *Clinical Handbook of Internal Medicine*, Volume 1, fifth printing, University of Western Sydney, Sydney, 2008.

- **SP-9** and **CV-12** resolve Dampness (foggy head, general heaviness of the body).
- **LU-10** clears Lung-Heat. Use when having no voice.
- **LU-11** expels Wind-Heat. Add if there is an extremely sore throat.
- **LI-20** and Yintang expel Wind-Heat and open the nose.
- **ST-25** can be used for abdominal distension or loose stools and **PC-6** for nausea.
- **SP-6** and **ST-36** support the Spleen, general tonification and immunity and resolve Dampness.

● Clinical Notes

- **SP-9** is the most essential point to resolve Dampness.

● Food

Avoid cow's milk, sugar, peanuts, bananas, fats and oils.

4 Wind-Dryness

This pattern might occur in very dry climates, in a dry centrally heated surrounding,[52] in a place with climate-control[53] or after an attack of Wind-Heat.[54]

● Clinical Signs and Symptoms

- Nasal congestion, dry mucosa
- Dry mouth, lips and throat
- Dry cough with little or no mucus
- Slight sweating
- Mild fever
- Aversion to wind and cold
- Headache.

---

52 Maciocia, G., *The Practice of Chinese Medicine: The Treatment of Diseases with Acupuncture and Chinese Herbs*, Churchill Livingstone, Edinburgh, 1994.
53 Own clinical expertise.
54 Maclean, W. and Lyttleton, J., *Clinical Handbook of Internal Medicine*, Volume 1, fifth printing, University of Western Sydney, Sydney, 2008.

Pulse: Floating (*Fu*), Wiry (*Xian*) and possibly Rapid (*Shuo*).

Tongue: Dry, slightly red and a thin white coating.

Season: Wind-Dryness is often seen in autumn.

- Treatment Principle
    - Expel Wind-Dryness.
    - Promote the descending and diffusing of Lung-Qi.
    - Moisten Dryness.
    - Open the nose.

- Acupuncture Points (select from)
LI-4 Hegu, **TB-5** Waiguan, **LI-11** Quchi, **LU-7** Lieque, **BL-12** Fengmen, **BL-13** Feishu, **LU-5** Chize, **LU-10** Yuji, **KI-6** Zhaohai, **LI-20** Yingxiang, **GB-20** Fengchi, **M-HN-3** Yintang, **SP-6** Sanyinjiao, **ST-36** Zusanli.

- Explanation
    - **LI-4**, **TB-5** and **LI-11** expel Wind-Heat and release the exterior.
    - **LU-7**, **BL-12** and **BL-13** promote the descending and diffusing of Lung-Qi (cough). Use **BL-12** in the early stage of the condition and **BL-13** for recurring pathology.
    - **LU-5** and **LU-10** (sore throat) clear Heat from the Lung.
    - **KI-6** nourishes Jin Ye, moistens Dryness and benefits the throat (dry throat, dry cough).
    - **LI-20** and Yintang expel Wind and open the nose.
    - **GB-20** eliminates Wind from the head. Add if there is a headache.
    - **SP-6** and **ST-36** support general tonification and immunity.

- Food
Pear juice.[55]

---

[55] Maclean, W. and Lyttleton, J., *Clinical Handbook of Internal Medicine*, Volume 1, fifth printing, University of Western Sydney, Sydney, 2008.

5 Wind-Cold with Internal Heat

Wind-Cold with internal Heat is often seen with smokers.[56] This is important to know as there are unfortunately many divers who smoke.

The exterior Wind-Cold attack combined with internal Heat can occur when there is already internal Heat.[57]

● Clinical Signs and Symptoms

- Thirst, wanting cold drinks
- Irritability and restlessness
- Sore throat
- Cough with sticky yellow sputum
- Nasal congestion
- High fever with chills
- No sweating
- Aversion to wind and cold
- Body aches
- Occipital headache and stiff neck
- Dry stools or constipation.

Pulse: Floating (*Fu*), Tight (*Jin*) and eventually Rapid (*Shuo*).

Tongue: Red or with a red tip and edges, a thin white or yellow coating.

● Treatment Principle

− Expel Wind-Cold and clear internal Heat.

− Promote the descending and diffusing of Lung-Qi.

− Open the nose.

● Acupuncture Points (select from)

LI-4 Hegu, **LU-7** Lieque, **TB-5** Waiguan, **LI-11** Quchi, **TB-2** Yemen, **BL-12** Fengmen, **BL-13** Feishu, **LI-20** Yingxiang, **GB-20** Fengchi, **M-HN-3** Yintang, **SP-6** Sanyinjiao, **ST-36** Zusanli.

---

56 Maclean, W. and Lyttleton, J., *Clinical Handbook of Internal Medicine*, Volume 1, fifth printing, University of Western Sydney, Sydney, 2008.
57 Sionneau, P. and Gang, L., *The Treatment of Disease in TCM, Volume 7: General Symptoms*, Blue Poppy Press, Boulder, CO, 2000.

- Explanation
    - **LI-4**, **LU-7** and **TB-5** clear Wind-Cold and release the exterior.
    - **LI-11** and **TB-2** clear internal Heat (fever, thirst).
    - **LU-7**, **BL-12** and **BL-13** promote the descending and diffusing of Lung-Qi (cough). Use **BL-12** in the early stage of the condition and **BL-13** for recurring pathology.
    - **LI-20** and Yintang expel Wind and open the nose.
    - **GB-20** eliminates Wind. Add in the case of blocked ears, a stiff neck or occipital headache.
    - **SP-6** and **ST-36** support general tonification and immunity.

- Food

First, take fresh ginger tea to release the exterior, and then cool internal Heat with pears, oranges, tangerines.

Advice for the Diver

It is strongly recommended *not* to dive with a common cold as there is a big chance of equalization problems! Take rest and only start diving when the common cold has disappeared totally.

1.7 RHINOSINUSITIS
鼻窦炎
Western Medicine
Definition and Aetiology

Rhinosinusitis is an inflammation of the mucosa in the sinuses *and* nasal cavity due to infection by bacteria or viruses, triggered by hyperreactivity of the mucosa or an allergy.

The sinuses consist of the frontal sinuses, ethmoidal sinuses (also called ethmoidal cells), sphenoidal sinuses and maxillary sinuses.

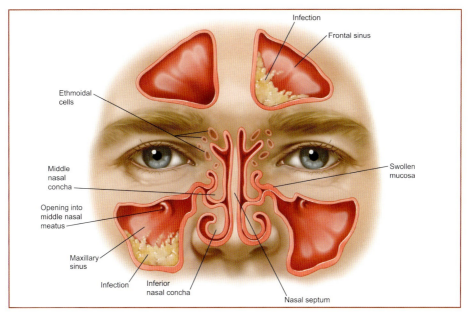

Figure 1.7.1 Rhinosinusitis

The name *sinusitis* changed to *rhinosinusitis* in the Netherlands in 2005 according the NHG-Standard (Standard for General Physicians) 'Rhinosinusitis, Second Revision' because 'the mucosa from the sinuses and the ostiomeatal complex are a continuum with the mucosa of the nose'.[58] When there is an inflammation the entire mucosa lining in nose, ostiomeatal complex and sinuses will be involved. Rhinosinusitis is the same as the ancient Chinese expression *Bi Yuan*, which is related 'with infection and inflammation of the sinuses and nasal cavity'.[59] It appears that Chinese physicians from centuries ago were innovative with their medical terminology already!

The revised NHG-Standard 'Acute Rhinosinusitis, Third Revision' (2014) says in summary:

> The mucosa from the nose are a continuum with the mucosa of the ostiomeatal complex and the mucosa of the sinuses. The ostiomeatal complex is the common drainage and ventilation place of the maxillary, frontal and anterior ethmoidal sinuses. Therefore, in the case of rhinosinusitis, except the maxillary sinus, the other sinuses are often inflamed as well. The complex is located below the middle turbinates and has an intricate and narrow construction. Swelling of the mucosa in this complex causes an obstruction

---

58 De Sutter, A., Burgers, J.S., De Bock, G.H., Dagnelie, C.F. *et al.*, 'NHG-Standaard Rhinosinusitis (Tweede herziening)', *Huisarts Wet* (2005) 48, 12, 615–626.
59 Maclean, W. and Lyttleton, J., *Clinical Handbook of Internal Medicine*, Volume 1, fifth printing, University of Western Sydney, Sydney, 2008 (p.234).

of the ostium by which the ventilation and clearing decreases and a breeding ground for micro-organisms can arise. Obstruction of the sinuses may cause pain or pressure in the face.[60]

According to this standard the diagnosis is made based on presenting symptoms: rhinorrhoea or congestion and at least one more symptom in the nose or sinuses such as anosmia and pain or pressure in the face.

Acute rhinosinusitis is caused by viruses associated with the common cold and flu and by bacteria. The most common viruses are rhinovirus, adenovirus, parainfluenza virus and influenza virus. The most common bacteria are Streptococcus pneumonia, Haemophilus influenza, Staphylococcus aureus and Moraxella catarrhalis. Acute rhinosinusitis often heals in ten days by itself but can last for four weeks.

Chronic rhinosinusitis has a duration of more than 12 weeks. The clinical signs and symptoms are somewhat more mild and common than in acute rhinosinusitis.

Sometimes I see divers after surgery (e.g. to widen the central duct of the maxillary sinus) who feel they have the same complaints as before the surgery. This is not the case as a couple of treatments are enough to get rid of the mucus, or sometimes a hematoma caused by the surgery and/or to calm the mucosa. Then the problem is totally solved and the effect of the surgery is there: no relapse.

Sinus Barotrauma

The sinuses clear automatically if there are no obstructions. The frontonasal canal (or frontal recess) is very long and narrow and due to its shape the frontal sinuses can be more complicated to equalize, in particular when there are swollen mucosa or phlegm. Therefore barotrauma of the frontal sinus occurs more frequently than of the maxillary sinus.

When pressure equalization is not possible due to a blockage in the osteomeatal complex there will be underpressure (vacuum) in the sinus during the descent (*squeeze*) or overpressure (expansion of air) during the ascent (*reverse block*). This can cause a very dangerous situation.

The frontal sinus squeeze and a reverse block can be accompanied by stabbing pain in the forehead, damage of the mucosa and blood coming out of the nose or mouth (there may be some blood in the mask). In the case of a reverse block it might be (almost) impossible to get back to the water surface due to extreme pain.

When they have an inflammation in the frontal sinus people are normally already in so much pain and feel ill in general that diving is not possible, and it is

---

60 Venekamp, R.P., De Sutter, A., Sachs, A., Bons, S.C.S., Wiersma, Tj and De Jongh, E. 'NHG-Standaard Acute rhinosinusitis (Derde herziening)', *Huisarts Wet* (2014) 57, 10, 537.

also strongly discouraged because of high barotrauma risks. A Dutch ENT doctor has said that these patients 'walk on their knees' to the hospital due to the intense pain. More frequently seen is an inflammation in the maxillary sinus.

Mucus Production and the Eustachian Tube

Some major facts about mucus production and the functions of the Eustachian tube:

- Normal mucus production from the nose, sinuses, Eustachian tube and middle ear is about one litre mucus per day of which half evaporates.[61]

- The Eustachian tube opens about once a minute when awake and about once every five minutes during sleep.[62]

- The opening time of the Eustachian tube is 0.1–0.6 seconds.[63]

- The function of the Eustachian tube is ventilation, drainage and protecting the middle ear against reflux, organisms, sound and air pressure changes in the pharynx.[64]

Diagnosis

The clinical signs and symptoms of rhinosinusitis are:

- nasal congestion or rhinorrhoea (discharge)
- anosmia (reduced sense of smell or no smell)
- postnasal drip (excess of phlegm from the nose that runs down the throat)
- cough
- sneezing
- slight or high fever
- headache

---

61 Brandt Corstius, J.J., Dermout, S.M. and Feenstra, L., *Duikgeneeskunde, Theorie en Praktijk*, tweede druk, Elsevier, Amsterdam, 2007.
62 Brandt Corstius, J.J., Dermout, S.M. and Feenstra, L., *Duikgeneeskunde, Theorie en Praktijk*, tweede druk, Elsevier, Amsterdam, 2007.
63 Brandt Corstius, J.J., Dermout, S.M. and Feenstra, L., *Duikgeneeskunde, Theorie en Praktijk*, tweede druk, Elsevier, Amsterdam, 2007.
64 Sehhati-Chafai-Leuwer, S., Wenzel, S., Bschorer, R., Seedorf, H., Kucinski, T. *et al.*, 'Pathophysiology of the Eustachian tube: Relevant new aspects for the head and neck surgeon', *Journal of Cranio-Maxillofacial Surgery* (2006) 34, 6, 351–354.

- facial pain, pain in forehead or maxillary sinus(es) when bending
- toothache, pain in the upper teeth and/or molars when chewing.

When someone has a dirty smelly nose there is an anaerobic (bacterial) inflammation and antibiotics might be needed. Most of the time the inflammation is secondary to a common cold or an allergic rhinopathy and often has a recurrent character.

Jaw rinses are not done any more because they are only a temporary solution. The openings close again.

Chronic rhinosinusitis is the most common chronic condition seen in the USA today and affects 37 million Americans a year.[65] Chinese medicine, including improving general health, supporting the immune system, preventing common cold and flus, reducing stress and improving daily food intake habits, might be the solution to reducing the occurrence of chronic rhinosinusitis, as well as treating the present clinical signs and symptoms (reducing phlegm, swollen mucosa, pain, etc.). In general lots of people use too much sugar, fats, cow's milk and alcohol and, unfortunately, refined sugars and flavours (E-numbers) are added in so many food products, which should not be necessary at all but contribute to illness and allergies.

Treatment

- Decongestion: nose drops/spray and pseudoephedrine (Sudafed®) oral tablets.
- Rinse with sodium chloride (salt).
- Painkillers: paracetamol or NSAIDs (like ibuprofen and naproxen).
- In acute rhinosinusitis antibiotics are generally not indicated as the positive effects on the complaints are very limited. Antibiotics are usually prescribed when people are really ill, when people have a reduced resistance to prevent complications, or when there has been a fever for more than five days or a fever comes back after a couple of fever-free days, in which case it's likely that a viral initial stage has developed into a bacterial inflammation (but the effect of the antibiotics in acute rhinosinusitis has not been scientifically proven). Antibiotics have side-effects such as weakening the intestinal flora and causing resistance, and that's why there is a more cautious policy currently regarding the prescription of antibiotics.[66]

---

65 Levine, H. and Rabago, D., 'Balloon sinuplasty: A minimally invasive option for patients with chronic rhinosinusitis', *Postgraduate Medicine* (2011) 123, 2, 112–118.

66 Venekamp, R.P., De Sutter, A., Sachs, A., Bons, S.C.S., Wiersma, Tj and De Jongh, E., 'NHG-Standaard Acute rhinosinusitis (Derde herziening)', *Huisarts Wet* (2014) 57, 10, 537.

- Clinical signs and symptoms of chronic or recurrent rhinosinusitis are usually mild, but the condition can develop into acute rhinosinusitis, in which case antibiotics will be prescribed.

- Surgery in chronic or recurrent rhinosinusitis: for example restoring the natural ostium (cutting or removal of bone/tissue) by widening the central gap of the sinus maxillary so the mucus can follow the movement of the cilia, which goes in direction of the central gap. In the past a lower gap was made in the sinus maxillary and the idea was that the phlegm could sink to the gap due to gravitation. The phlegm unfortunately did not go that way because the cilia push the phlegm in the direction of the natural central gap. This last surgery technique has been done for about ten years without any result.

- Balloon sinuplasty in chronic or recurrent rhinosinusitis. This relatively new (2005) and less invasive technique (no cutting or removal of bone/tissue) consists of several steps:
  - inserting a latex-free balloon catheter into the inflamed sinus
  - inflating the balloon to widen the ductus
  - bringing in saline (sodium chloride) to rinse the sinus
  - removing the balloon catheter, resulting in a restructured ductus (associated risks: trauma of mucosa/tissue, infection and possibly optic injury;[67] but these risks can occur with traditional sinus surgery as well).

Chinese Medicine
Definition and Aetiology

Bi Yuan (rhinosinusitis) means there is an infection or inflammation in the sinuses and nasal cavities. When there is an inflammation, the mucous glands in the sinuses secrete more mucus, which can obstruct the nose and sinuses.

Bi Zhi (nasal congestion) refers to chronic nasal congestion that can exist 'with or without infection'.[68]

Generally rhinosinusitis and nasal congestion can be divided into:

---

67 Acclarent, 'Sinus Surgery with Balloon Sinuplasty', Balloon Sinuplasty, www.balloonsinuplasty.com/what-is-balloon-sinuplasty/procedure-overview (accessed 8 August 2017).

68 Maclean, W. and Lyttleton, J., *Clinical Handbook of Internal Medicine*, Volume 1, fifth printing, University of Western Sydney, Sydney, 2008 (p.234).

- acute pathology due to invasions of Wind-Cold and Wind-Heat, which can result in Lung-Heat, and due to improper diet resulting in Phlegm-Heat (which might develop into chronic Phlegm-Heat)

- chronic pathology with Liver-Qi Stagnation/Heat, leading to Liver and Gall Bladder-Fire and deficiency of the Lung-Qi, the Spleen-Qi and the Kidney.[69]

All chronic constitutions may result in stagnation of Qi and Xue.

People who suffer from recurrent or chronic rhinosinusitis generally have a weak immune system, or an overactive immune system always working to overcome some pathogen in the sinuses. Often there is an underlying organ deficiency making the Wei Qi less strong, and people can develop chronic nasal congestion and discharge easily. The discharge is often Phlegm due to deficiency of the Lung, Spleen, Kidney or as a result of Liver-Qi stagnation, and there is not always an infection.

Acute rhinosinusitis is often the result of a secondary bacterial infection due to a poor recovery from a common cold or flu, allergic rhinitis, a viral upper respiratory tract infection and sometimes dental infection.

Stress, worries, improper diet, antibiotics and not taking enough rest are commonly seen issues in our modern society where people have too busy agendas, which can lead to deficiencies of the organs and the production of Phlegm.

BOX 1.7.1 ANTIBIOTICS

Antibiotics clear Heat but don't resolve Dampness, which can cause long-term problems in the sinuses. Dampness and Phlegm can remain in the sinuses and create an ideal condition for recurrent Phlegm-Heat.[70]

BOX 1.7.2 THE SINUSES AND THE EFFECTS OF THE ACUPUNCTURE POINTS

I want to emphasize that in almost all standard literature about Chinese medicine only the frontal and maxillary sinuses are mentioned regarding sinus pathology and extra points treating the sinuses. Surprisingly the *ethmoidal* and *sphenoidal sinuses* are rarely noted.

---

69 Maclean, W. and Lyttleton, J., *Clinical Handbook of Internal Medicine*, Volume 1, fifth printing, University of Western Sydney, Sydney, 2008.
70 Maclean, W. and Lyttleton, J., *Clinical Handbook of Internal Medicine*, Volume 1, fifth printing, University of Western Sydney, Sydney, 2008.

EAR, NOSE AND THROAT DISORDERS

When showing clinical signs and symptoms of pain and/or swelling in between the eyes, or swelling of the eyelids, it may imply that the ethmoidal sinuses are inflamed. When there is ear pain, neck pain or deep pain of the top of the head, it is possible that the sphenoidal sinuses are affected. Inflammation in the sphenoidal sinuses is less common but can be dangerous, being located close to the pituitary gland (*hypophysis*). An X-ray, MRI or CT scan is needed to diagnose which sinus(es) is (are) affected.

Bearing in mind the meaning of rhinosinusitis (as noted above, the mucosa of the sinuses and the ostiomeatal complex are a continuum with the mucosa of the nose), the functions of **M-HN-3** Yintang, **(EX)** Biyan, **M-HN-14** Bitong and **M-HN-6** Yuyao *and* their location, it is very plausible that these extra points influence the ethmoidal and sphenoidal sinuses as well.

Channels: The Bladder and Gall Bladder channels affect the frontal, ethmoidal and sphenoidal sinuses. The Stomach, Large Intestine and Small Intestine channels influence the maxillary sinuses.[71]

Table 1.7.1 Essential acupuncture points to benefit the nose and sinuses

Nose	Frontal sinus	Maxillary sinus
LI-20 Yingxiang	**BL-2** Zanzhu	**LI-20** Yingxiang
BL-2 Zanzhu	**GB-14** Yangbai	**ST-3** Juliao
LI-4 Hegu	**GV-23** Shangxing	**ST-2** Sibai
LU-7 Lieque	**M-HN-3** Yintang	**GV-23** Shangxing
GB-39 Xuanzhong	**M-HN-6** Yuyao	**M-HN-14** Bitong
GV-23 Shangxing	**M-HN-9** Taiyang	**M-HN-9** Taiyang
M-HN-3 Yintang		Wrist Point 1
M-HN-14 Bitong		
(EX) Biyan		
YNSA Nose Point		
Wrist Point 1		

---

71 Diamond, J., *The Clinical Practice of Complementary, Alternative, and Western Medicine*, CRC Press LLC, Boca Raton, FL, 2001.

Table 1.7.2 Acupuncture points to reduce Dampness and Phlegm in case of ENT disorders. Use depending on the existing Chinese medical diagnosis

Dampness	Phlegm
SP-9 Yinlingquan	**ST-40** Fenglong
SP-6 Sanjinyiao	**ST-36** Zusanli
SP-3 Taibai (Dampness and Damp-Heat)	**CV-12** Zhongwan (postnasal drip)
SP-4 Gongsun	
CV-12 Zhongwan	
ST-40 Fenglong	
TB-5 Waiguan (External Damp pathogens)	
LI-11 Quchi	
BL-20 Pishu	
GB-34 Yanglingquan (Damp-Heat Gall Bladder organ)	
GB-43 Xiaxi (Damp-Heat Gall Bladder channel)	

(EX) Biyan, M-HN-14 Bitong and YNSA Nose Point

In chronic nasal obstruction that is very hard to influence the Chinese extra point Biyan (*Eyes of Nose*) and the Nose Point according to Yamamoto New Scalp Acupuncture (YNSA) (see the section 'YNSA Sensory Points' below) give great results.

For the extra point Biyan, which I learned about at the Nanchang Hospital in China in 1994 and at Jing Ming College in Belgium (1991–1994), no **M-HN** number is available. That's why I have decided to add **(EX)** to distinguish it from other point numbering. **(EX)** Biyan especially affects the nose but supports the treatment of sinus disorders as well.

I prefer **(EX)** Biyan to **M-HN-14** Bitong when the nose is very obstructed due to dry mucous membranes. **(EX)** Biyan is not a very well known point but is very effective, in particular when the obstruction is hard to break through. I usually choose **M-HN-14** Bitong for a clogged tear duct or problems with the maxillary sinus (where the point is usually swollen).

*Location of **(EX)** Biyan:* Lateral to the midline and midpoint of the nose, between the bone and cartilage of the nose.

*Location of **M-HN-14** Bitong:* At the highest point of the nasolabial groove.

EAR, NOSE AND THROAT DISORDERS

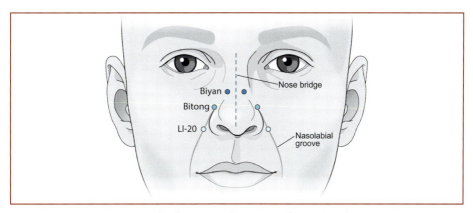

Figure 1.7.2 Extra Points **(EX)** Biyan and **M-HN-14** (Bitong) with **LI-20** Yingxiang

YNSA Sensory Points

To treat ENT disorders with YNSA sensory points combined with the traditional points, it is most practical to use the points located at the anterior (Yin) side of the head (see Figure 1.7.3) as the YNSA points are situated at the posterior (Yang) side as well. The YNSA sensory points are the Eye, Nose, Mouth and Ear Points.

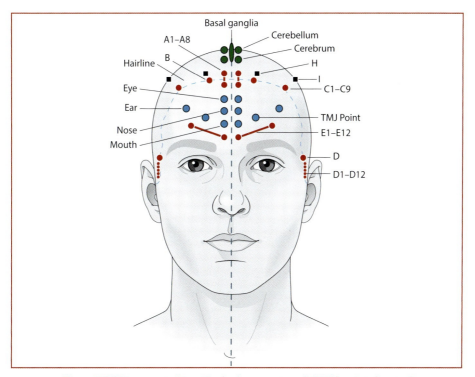

Figure 1.7.3 Yamamoto New Scalp Acupuncture (YNSA) points located at the anterior side (Yin) of the head. The TMJ Point was located and described by Dr R.A. Feely, who studied with Dr Yamamoto

The *Eye Point* benefits all eye disorders. In ENT disorders accompanied by eye problems this point can be used as well as the traditional points (e.g. for allergic conjunctivitis, severe lacrimation, dryness or pain of the eyes).

Location: Approximately 1 cm bilateral from the midline and about 1 cm distal from the most inferior Basic A Point.[72]

The *Nose Point* is effective in all nose and sinus disorders (nasal congestion, anosmia, rhinosinusitis, allergic rhinitis, posttraumatic and postoperative pain).

Location: Approximately 1 cm bilateral from the midline and about 1 cm inferior from the Eye Point.[73]

The *Mouth Point* is useful for all mouth disorders (tonsillitis, pharyngitis, TMJ disorder).

Location: Approximately 1 cm bilateral from the midline and about 1 cm inferior from the Nose Point.[74]

The *Ear Point* is effective in all ear disorders (like otitis, tinnitus, posttraumatic and postoperative pain).

Location: Approximately 1.5 cm inferior from the Basic C Point on a 45-degree line between the C Point and the root of the nose.[75]

> ### BOX 1.7.3 YAMAMOTO NEW SCALP ACUPUNCTURE (YNSA)
>
> Yamamoto New Scalp Acupuncture, developed by Japanese physician Toshikatsu Yamamoto, is a microsystem based on reflexology of the kinetic apparatus, the sensory and internal organs and the brain. The size of the YNSA points is approximately 1 mm.[76] When there is pathology the YNSA points are painful on palpation and can have properties like resistance, hardness, softness, swelling or an indentation and superficial redness or scaling of the skin.[77] Needling a disturbed YNSA point is accompanied by a strong sensation at the scalp.

----

72 Yamamoto, T. and Yamamoto, H., *Yamamoto New Scalp Acupuncture: YNSA*, Medical Tribune Inc., Tokyo, 2006.
73 Yamamoto, T. and Yamamoto, H., *Yamamoto New Scalp Acupuncture: YNSA*, Medical Tribune Inc., Tokyo, 2006.
74 Yamamoto, T. and Yamamoto, H., *Yamamoto New Scalp Acupuncture: YNSA*, Medical Tribune Inc., Tokyo, 2006.
75 Yamamoto, T. and Yamamoto, H., *Yamamoto New Scalp Acupuncture: YNSA*, Medical Tribune Inc., Tokyo, 2006.
76 Yamamoto, T. and Yamamoto, H., *Yamamoto New Scalp Acupuncture: YNSA*, Medical Tribune Inc., Tokyo, 2006.
77 Yamamoto, T. and Yamamoto, H., *Yamamoto New Scalp Acupuncture: YNSA*, Medical Tribune Inc., Tokyo, 2006.

EAR, NOSE AND THROAT DISORDERS

Wrist-Ankle Acupuncture

It also might be helpful to use *Wrist Point 1* (*Upper 1*) from 'wrist-ankle acupuncture', developed by Dr Zhang Xinshu and his colleagues Zhou Qinghui and Ling Changquan. Wrist-ankle acupuncture is based on reflexology, which I learned to use while studying at the China Beijing International Acupuncture Training Centre in 2004.

Upper 1 is useful in a common cold, allergic rhinitis, hyperreactive rhinitis, rhinosinusitis, pharyngitis, tonsillitis, cough, chills and fever.[78, 79]

I like to add Wrist Point 1 to my point selection in chronic nasal obstruction (when the obstruction is very difficult to break through), but the point can be used in acute situations as well.

Location: 2 CUN proximal to the transverse crease of the wrist, on the palmar/ulnar side, in between the ulna and the tendon of the flexor carpi ulnaris muscle.[80]

An interesting point from this wrist-ankle method to mention in this book – useful in ear and TMJ pathology – is *Wrist Point 4* (*Upper 4*). Wrist Point 4 is helpful in ear pain, tinnitus, hearing loss and TMJ disorders.[81]

Location: 2 CUN proximal to the transverse crease of the wrist, on the lateral border of the radius at the juncture of the palmar and dorsal side.[82]

Needling Technique for Wrist Points

- It is preferable to use needles 0.25 mm x 25 mm in length ('Gauge 32 and 1.0 CUN (inch)'[83]).

- Needle subcutaneously and slowly (like needling **LU-7**), with an angle of 30 degrees.

- Needle in proximal direction in ENT and TMJ disorders.

- The subcutaneous needle insertion may not have any needle sensation. The insertion should be painfree as the subcutaneous layer is poorly innervated.

....

78 Dai, C.Y., Lecture: 'Wrist-Ankle Acupuncture', China Beijing International Acupuncture Training Centre, 2004.
79 Zhou, Q.G., Ling, C.Q. and Zhang, X.S., *Wrist-Ankle Acupuncture*, Publishing House of Shanghai University of Traditional Chinese Medicine, Shanghai, 2002.
80 Zhou, Q.G., Ling, C.Q. and Zhang, X.S., *Wrist-Ankle Acupuncture*, Publishing House of Shanghai University of Traditional Chinese Medicine, Shanghai, 2002.
81 Zhou, Q.G., Ling, C.Q. and Zhang, X.S., *Wrist-Ankle Acupuncture*, Publishing House of Shanghai University of Traditional Chinese Medicine, Shanghai, 2002.
82 Zhou, Q.G., Ling, C.Q. and Zhang, X.S., *Wrist-Ankle Acupuncture*, Publishing House of Shanghai University of Traditional Chinese Medicine, Shanghai, 2002.
83 Zhou, Q.G., Ling, C.Q. and Zhang, X.S., *Wrist-Ankle Acupuncture*, Publishing House of Shanghai University of Traditional Chinese Medicine, Shanghai, 2002 (p.27).

- You can feel the needle under the skin.
- Needle retention time: at least 30 minutes.

Pattern Differentiation: Acute Rhinosinusitis
1 Wind-Cold
An invasion of Wind-Cold can occur due to weakness of Wei Qi, when the pathogenic factor is very strong or if there is not sufficient external body protection (see Section 1.6). Wind-Cold constricts the flow of Lung-Qi, thereby blocking the distribution of Jin Ye in the nose and sinuses, whereby they stagnate and congeal into Phlegm. Subsequently Wind-Cold can transform into Wind-Heat.

● Clinical Signs and Symptoms
- Nasal congestion or clear or white watery discharge
- Inflamed and swollen mucous membranes
- Anosmia
- Aversion to cold
- Contemporary fever and chills
- Body aches
- Occipital or frontal headache, maxillary pain.

Pulse: Floating (*Fu*) and Tight (*Jin*).

Tongue: Normal (in the initial stage) or with a thin white coating.

● Treatment Principle
- Expel Wind-Cold.
- Promote the descending and diffusing of Lung-Qi.
- Open the nose and sinuses.

● Acupuncture Points (select from)
LI-4 Hegu, **LU-7** Lieque, **TB-5** Waiguan, **LU-9** Taiyuan, **BL-12** Fengmen, **BL-13** Feishu, **LI-20** Yingxiang, **BL-2** Zanzhu, **ST-2** Sibai, **ST-3** Juliao, **GB-14** Yangbai, **GV-23** Shangxing, **M-HN-3** Yintang, **M-HN-6** Yuyao, **M-HN-9** Taiyang, **M-HN-14** Bitong, **(EX)** Biyan, YNSA Nose Point, **GB-20** Fengchi, **SP-6** Sanyinjiao, **ST-36** Zusanli.

EAR, NOSE AND THROAT DISORDERS

● Explanation

- **LI-4**, **LU-7** and **TB-5** expel Wind-Cold and release the exterior.
- **LU-7**, **LU-9**, **BL-12** and **BL-13** promote the descending and diffusing of Lung-Qi, which prevents accumulation of Jin Ye in the nose and sinuses. Use **BL-12** in the early stage of the condition and **BL-13** in recurring pathology.
- **LI-20**, **BL-2**, **ST-2**, **ST-3**, **GB-14**, **GV-23**, Yintang, Yuyao, Taiyang, Bitong and Biyan benefit the nose and/or sinuses (congestion, discharge, pain, sneezing, anosmia).
  - Choose local points depending on the affected zones (see Tables 1.7.3 and 1.7.4).
- YNSA Nose Point is a good addition when the nose is hard to open.
- **GB-20** eliminates Wind from the head. Use in blocked ears, a stiff neck or headache.
- **SP-6** and **ST-36** support general tonification and immunity.

● Clinical Notes

- **LU-9** is especially used for chronic patterns but I prefer to needle this point in combination with **LU-7** in acute situations as well (besides using this combination for chronic conditions). The points applied together fortify each other's actions whereby rhinosinusitis improves faster. I have learned to needle these points as a forceful combination from acupuncturist/teacher Bruno Braeckman while studying acupuncture in Belgium at Jing Ming College during 1991–1994.

Table 1.7.3 Local acupuncture points to influence ENT disorders

Acupuncture points	Affected zones
LI-20 Yingxiang	Nose, maxillary sinus
BL-2 Zanzhu	Nose, frontal sinus, eyes
ST-2 Sibai	Maxillary sinus, eyes
ST-3 Juliao	Maxillary sinus, external nose, cheek
GB-14 Yangbai	Frontal sinus, eyes
GV-23 Shangxing	Nose, frontal and maxillary sinus, eyes

Table 1.7.4 Extra points with the affected zones and needling direction

Extra points	Affected zones	Needling direction
M-HN-3 Yintang	Nose, frontal sinuses	Inferior direction
M-HN-6 Yuyao	Frontal sinus, eye, eyelid	Medial direction for frontal sinus
M-HN-9 Taiyang	Frontal, maxillary sinus	Inferior direction for maxillary sinus, medial direction for frontal sinus
M-HN-14 Bitong	Nose, maxillary sinus	Towards nose bridge
(EX) Biyan	Nose	Perpendicular direction

Note: Needling depth of these extra points is dependent on the location and the affected zone(s): in general between 0.1 and 1 CUN

2 Wind-Heat

Wind-Heat dries and damages Jin Ye, and blocks the descending and diffusing of Lung-Qi resulting in thickened and stagnant fluids in the nose and sinuses. Wind-Heat can transform into Lung-Heat.

● Clinical Signs and Symptoms

- Thick, sticky yellow or green discharge or nasal congestion
- Inflamed and swollen mucous membranes
- Fever, chills and thirst
- Cough with yellow sputum
- Anosmia
- Frontal headache or maxillary pain.

Pulse: Floating (*Fu*) and Rapid (*Shuo*).

Tongue: Normal (in the initial stage) or with a red front and/or a yellow coating.

● Treatment Principle

− Clear Wind-Heat.
− Promote the descending and diffusing of Lung-Qi.
− Open the nose and sinuses.

● Acupuncture Points (select from)

LI-4 Hegu, **LI-11** Quchi, **TB-5** Waiguan, **LU-5** Chize, **LU-10** Yuji, **LU-7** Lieque, **LU-9** Taiyuan, **BL-12** Fengmen, **BL-13** Feishu, **LI-20** Yingxiang, **BL-2** Zanzhu, **ST-2** Sibai, **ST-3** Juliao, **GB-14** Yangbai, **GV-23** Shangxing, **M-HN-3** Yintang, **M-HN-6** Yuyao, **M-HN-9** Taiyang, **M-HN-14** Bitong, **(EX)** Biyan,

YNSA Nose Point, **GB-20** Fengchi, **GV-14** Dazhui, **SP-6** Sanyinjiao, **ST-36** Zusanli.

● Explanation

- **LI-4**, **LI-11** and **TB-5** expel Wind-Heat and release the exterior.

- **LU-5** (cough) and **LU-10** (no voice) clear Heat from the Lung.

- **LU-7**, **LU-9**, **BL-12** and **BL-13** promote the descending and diffusing of Lung-Qi. Use **BL-12** in the early stage of the condition and **BL-13** in case of recurring pathology.

- **LI-20**, **BL-2**, **ST-2**, **ST-3**, **GB-14**, **GV-23**, Yintang, Yuyao, Taiyang, Bitong and Biyan benefit the nose and/or sinuses (congestion, discharge, pain, sneezing, anosmia).

    - Choose local points depending on the affected zones (see Tables 1.7.3 and 1.7.4).

- YNSA Nose Point is a good addition when the nose is hard to open.

- **GB-20** eliminates Wind from the head. Add in the case of headache.

- **GV-14** clears Heat. Use when there is fever.

- **SP-6** and **ST-36** support general tonification and immunity.

3 Phlegm-Heat

Phlegm-Heat can be caused by improper diet (greasy, fried and spicy food), alcohol or emotional stress (obsessive thinking), and might be a result of Wind-Heat. It can occur in an acute and chronic phase.

● Clinical Signs and Symptoms

- Sticky yellow or green nasal discharge, or marked nasal congestion
- Inflamed and swollen mucous membranes
- Heaviness of the head, foggy head
- Anosmia
- Frontal headache or maxillary pain
- Epigastric distension
- Thirst
- Tiredness.

Pulse: Slippery (*Hua*) and Rapid (*Shuo*).

Tongue: Red with a greasy yellow coating.

● Treatment Principle

- Clear and transform Phlegm-Heat.
- Promote the descending and diffusing of Lung-Qi.
- Open the nose and sinuses.

● Acupuncture Points (select from)

ST-40 Fenglong, **CV-12** Zhongwan, **LU-5** Chize, **LU-10** Yuji, **LI-11** Quchi, **LU-7** Lieque, **LU-9** Taiyuan, **LI-20** Yingxiang, **BL-2** Zanzhu, **ST-2** Sibai, **ST-3** Juliao, **GB-14** Yangbai, **GV-23** Shangxing, **M-HN-3** Yintang, **M-HN-6** Yuyao, **M-HN-9** Taiyang, **M-HN-14** Bitong, **(EX)** Biyan, YNSA Nose Point, **SP-3** Taibai, **SP-4** Gongsun, **SP-6** Sanyinjiao, **ST-36** Zusanli.

● Explanation

- **ST-40** and **CV-12** transform Phlegm. **CV-12** can be added in the case of postnasal drip.
- **LU-5**, **LU-10** and **LI-11** clear internal Heat (thirst).
- **LU-7** and **LU-9** promote the descending and diffusing of Lung-Qi.
- **LI-20**, **BL-2**, **ST-2**, **ST-3**, **GB-14**, **GV-23**, Yintang, Yuyao, Taiyang, Bitong and Biyan benefit the nose and/or sinuses (congestion, discharge, pain, anosmia, sneezing).
   - Choose local points depending on the affected zones (see Tables 1.7.3 and 1.7.4).
- YNSA Nose Point is a good addition when the nose is hard to open.
- **SP-3**, **SP-4** and **SP-6** strengthen the Spleen (important to prevent the onset of Phlegm).
- **ST-36** fortifies the Spleen, resolves Phlegm and supports the immunity.

● Clinical Notes

- **ST-40** is the most important point to transform Phlegm.
- To decrease postnasal drip **CV-12** is a very effective distal point.
- **GV-23** is mainly used in the case of chronic nose and sinus conditions.

EAR, NOSE AND THROAT DISORDERS

● Food

No cow's milk (goat's milk is okay), sugar, hot and greasy foods, alcohol and coffee. Grapefruit and pear have cooling properties and transform Phlegm.

If the patient is overweight, work with him or her to achieve a healthy weight and condition.

Advise to improve general health with good food and a variety in the meals.

> ### ⓘ BOX 1.7.4 ORIGIN OF PHLEGM
>
> The formation of Phlegm can be caused by:[84]
> - deficiency of the Lung or external Wind attacking the Lung
>   - ➔ impairment or obstruction of descending and diffusing of Jin Ye
>   - ➔ Jin Ye coagulate ➔ Phlegm
> - deficiency of the Spleen
>   - ➔ disharmony of transformation and transportation of Jin Ye
>   - ➔ Dampness ➔ Dampness stagnates ➔ Phlegm
> - deficiency of the Kidney
>   - ➔ stagnation of Jin Ye ➔ Phlegm
> - excess or deficient Heat
>   - ➔ Jin Ye condense ➔ Phlegm
> - Liver-Qi stagnation
>   - ➔ Fire ➔ Jin Ye congeal ➔ Phlegm
>
> #### Clinical Notes
>
> - During diving the dry and cold compressed air from the tank can irritate the mucous membranes and dry the Jin Ye of the throat, nose, sinuses and Eustachian tube, which may contribute to the development of Phlegm.[85]

> ### ⓘ BOX 1.7.5 JIN YE (BODY FLUIDS)
>
> Jin Ye are *Body Fluids* and originate from our food and drink (Gu Qi). The Jin Fluids are clear, light, watery, more active (Yang) than Ye Fluids and circulate with the Wei Qi at the exterior (moisten and nourish skin and muscles). The Ye Fluids are turbid and sticky, more slow (Yin) and circulate with the Ying Qi

---

[84] Adapted from Maciocia, G., *The Foundations of Chinese Medicine: A Comprehensive Text*, third edition, Elsevier, Amsterdam, 2015 and Deadman, P., Al-Khafaji, M. and Baker, K., *A Manual of Acupuncture*, Journal of Chinese Medicine Publications, Hove, 2015.

[85] Own clinical expertise.

> (Nutritive Qi) in the interior (moisten and nourish joints, spine, bone marrow and brain).
>
> Jin Fluids manifest as sweat (Heart), mucus (Lung), light watery saliva (Spleen), more thick viscous salvia (Kidney) and tears (Liver). Ye Fluids moisten and nourish the orifices of the sense organs (eyes, ears, nose and mouth).
>
> Disharmony of Jin Ye can result in Dampness or Phlegm.

Pattern Differentiation: Chronic Rhinosinusitis and Recurring Common Colds

The patterns for chronic rhinosinusitis (points 1–4) and recurring common colds (points 1–3) I treat the most in my practice regarding the underlying deficiency include:

1. Lung-Qi deficiency
2. Spleen-Qi deficiency
3. Kidney-Yin, Kidney-Yang and Kidney-Jing deficiency
4. Liver-Qi stagnation, leading to Liver and Gall Bladder-Fire.

Often there is a combination of deficiencies of the different organs. When the deficiency occurs over a long time the patterns may result in Qi and Xue stagnation, which may end up in Dryness in the nose and sinuses. The last situation takes more time to improve and recover totally and it is usually harder to open the nose when the mucosa are dry.

It's very important to treat the deficiency to strengthen the energy system, which supports the Wei Qi, because deficiency problems are very common with divers who have problems clearing the ears.

1 Lung-Qi Deficiency

Lung-Qi can be deficient due to congenital factors, sadness, grief, lots of talking, bad posture (sitting hunched causing superficial breathing), smoking and chronic or repetitive nose and/or sinus disorders.

● Clinical Signs and Symptoms

- Inoffensive thin white or sticky nasal discharge, or chronic nasal congestion, better in the day and worse when laying down/at night
- Anosmia
- Dyspnoea
- Weak voice

- Cough
- Tiredness
- Pale face
- Spontaneous sweating
- Dislike of cold.

Pulse: Deficient (*Xu*) or Weak (*Ruo*).

Tongue: Pale with a thin white coating.

● Treatment Principle

- Tonify Lung-Qi.
- Promote the descending and diffusing of Lung-Qi.
- Transform Phlegm.
- Open the nose and sinuses.

● Acupuncture Points (select from)
LU-7 Lieque, **LU-9** Taiyuan, **BL-13** Feishu, **LU-2** Yunmen, **CV-17** Shanzhong, **ST-40** Fenglong, **LI-20** Yingxiang, **BL-2** Zanzhu, **ST-2** Sibai, **ST-3** Juliao, **GB-14** Yangbai, **GV-23** Shangxing, **M-HN-3** Yintang, **M-HN-6** Yuyao, **M-HN-9** Taiyang, **M-HN-14** Bitong, **(EX)** Biyan, YNSA Nose Point, Wrist Point 1.

● Explanation

- **LU-7**, **LU-9** and **BL-13** tonify Lung-Qi and promote its descending and diffusion.
- **LU-2** and **CV-17** descend Lung-Qi. Use if there is dyspnoea, high sternal breathing, fullness in the chest and/or cough.
- **ST-40** transforms Phlegm.
- **LI-20**, **BL-2**, **ST-2**, **ST-3**, **GB-14**, **GV-23**, Yintang, Yuyao, Taiyang, Bitong and Biyan benefit the nose and/or sinuses (congestion, discharge, pain, anosmia, sneezing).
  - Choose local points depending on the affected zones (see Tables 1.7.3 and 1.7.4).
- YNSA Nose Point or Wrist Point 1 is a good addition when the nose is hard to open.

- Clinical Notes
    - **CV-17** is useful when there is a tendency to get common colds easily as it strengthens Zong Qi (Gathering Qi).

- Food

Asparagus. Tea from Bulbus Lilii (Bai He).

2 Spleen-Qi Deficiency

In Spleen-Qi deficiency there is often an emotional cause, such as overthinking, but it can also be the result of using or having used too many antibiotics, an irregular diet or a diet to lose weight. Eating too much sugar can decrease the Spleen-Qi and cause Phlegm.

Earth fails to support Metal in the generating (Sheng) cycle. The Liver can suppress the Spleen and diminish Spleen-Qi (e.g. when there is a lot of anger). Weak Spleen-Qi can lead to chronic Phlegm-Heat as well and in that case the mucus is sticky and yellow and the pulse will be Slippery (*Hua*) and Rapid (*Shuo*).

- Clinical Signs and Symptoms
    - Chronic sticky, white nasal discharge or nasal congestion, which is better in the daytime
    - Pale and swollen mucous membranes
    - Anosmia
    - Fuzziness of the head
    - Heaviness of the body
    - Tiredness especially in the morning (starting problems)
    - Borborygmus (intestinal rumblings)
    - Poor appetite
    - Distension of the abdomen, loose stools
    - Tendency to be overweight (especially the belly region)
    - Obsessive thinking.

Pulse: Deficient (*Xu*) or Weak (*Ruo*).

In the case of Dampness and Phlegm due to Spleen deficiency the pulse is Slippery (*Hua*); Dampness due to weak Spleen deficiency can be felt as Soggy (*Ru*) as well.

Tongue: Pale, swollen and tooth marks.

- Treatment Principle
    - Tonify Spleen-Qi.
    - Transform Damp and its resultant Phlegm.
    - Open the nose and sinuses.

- Acupuncture Points (select from)
SP-6 Sanyinjiao, **SP-4** Gongsun, **SP-3** Taibai, **BL-20** Pishu, **SP-9** Yinlingquan, **CV-12** Zhongwan, **ST-36** Zusanli, **ST-40** Fenglong, **LI-20** Yingxiang, **BL-2** Zanzhu, **ST-2** Sibai, **ST-3** Juliao, **GB-14** Yangbai, **GV-23** Shangxing, **M-HN-3** Yintang, **M-HN-6** Yuyao, **M-HN-9** Taiyang, **M-HN-14** Bitong, **(EX)** Biyan, YNSA Nose Point, Wrist Point 1.

- Explanation
    - **SP-6**, **SP-4**, **SP-3** and **BL-20** tonify Spleen-Qi and resolve Dampness.
    - **SP-9** and **CV-12** resolve Dampness.
    - **ST-36** fortifies the Spleen, resolves Dampness and Phlegm, supports the immunity.
    - **ST-40** transforms Phlegm.
    - **LI-20**, **BL-2**, **ST-2**, **ST-3**, **GB-14**, **GV-23**, Yintang, Yuyao, Taiyang, Bitong and Biyan benefit the nose and/or sinuses (congestion, discharge, pain, anosmia, sneezing).
        - Choose local points depending on the affected zones (see Tables 1.7.3 and 1.7.4).
    - YNSA Nose Point or Wrist Point 1 is a good addition when the nose is hard to open.

- Food
No (not too much) sugar and no cold foods. Beneficial are cooked and warm foods, corn, rice, oats, spelt, sweet potato. Coffee dries Dampness and stimulates the brain (maximum of 1–2 cups per day).

3 Kidney Deficiency
The underlying Kidney-Yin and Kidney-Yang problems are chronic patterns due to congenital problems, a busy lifestyle (no rest), hormonal disbalance, excessive sexual activity (depletes especially Jing), loss of Jin Ye and/or Xue (Kidney-Yin deficiency) or a chronic disease.

When Kidney-Yin is injured, Kidney-Yang will regularly become deficient as well and vice versa. Regarding the treatment of Kidney-Yin deficiency, it's important to treat Kidney-Yang also because it will nourish Kidney-Yin (and treating Kidney-Yin will fortify Kidney-Yang). Therefore both Kidney-Yin and Kidney-Yang are nourished and tonified by most Kidney points.[86]

- Kidney-Yin Deficiency: Clinical Signs and Symptoms
    - Chronic nasal congestion, dry mucosa
    - Anosmia
    - Mild sore throat with dryness
    - Concentration problems, blurred vision
    - Flushing in the face
    - Night sweating (Five-palm Heat; this is a feeling of heat in the palms of the hands, soles of the feet, and chest)
    - Tiredness
    - Headache and/or dizziness
    - Tinnitus
    - Aching and weakness in the lower back and knees.

Pulse: Thready (*Xi*) and Rapid (*Shuo*).

Tongue: Red and dry with a slight yellow or no coating.

- Kidney-Yang Deficiency: Clinical Signs and Symptoms
    - Chronic nasal watery discharge or nasal congestion
    - Anosmia
    - Pale complexion
    - Coldness, soreness and weakness in lower back and knees, cold intolerance
    - Hearing loss, deafness
    - Low libido, impotence, infertility due to coldness in the uterus
    - Concentration problems

---

86 Deadman, P., Al-Khafaji, M. and Baker, K., *A Manual of Acupuncture,* Journal of Chinese Medicine Publications, Hove, 2015.

- Tiredness
- Lethargy (no will to do something)
- Frequent urination in the night with copious clear urine.

Pulse: Deep (*Chen*), Thready (*Xi*) and Slow (*Chi*).

Tongue: Pale and swollen with a white coating.

● Kidney-Jing Deficiency: Clinical Signs and Symptoms

- Soreness and weakness in the lower back and knees
- Tinnitus, deafness
- Blurred vision
- Infertility, low libido
- Falling or (premature) greying hair
- Loose teeth
- Bone problems (development, softening)
- Forgetfulness and poor memory.

There may be no specific Hot or Cold signs if Kidney-Yin and Kidney-Yang are equally weak.

Pulse: Deep (*Chen*), Thready (*Xi*) and Weak (*Ruo*).

Tongue: Variable with more deficient Yin or Yang.

● Treatment Principle

- Nourish and tonify Kidney-Yin, Kidney-Yang and/or Kidney-Jing.
- Open the nose and sinuses.
- Transform Phlegm.

● Acupuncture Points (select from)

KI-3 Taixi, **KI-6** Zhaohai, **CV-4** Guanyuan, **CV-6** Qihai, **GV-4** Mingmen, **BL-23** Shenshu, **ST-40** Fenglong, **LI-20** Yingxiang, **BL-2** Zanzhu, **ST-2** Sibai, **ST-3** Juliao, **GB-14** Yangbai, **GV-23** Shangxing, **M-HN-3** Yintang, **M-HN-6** Yuyao, **M-HN-9** Taiyang, **M-HN-14** Bitong, **(EX)** Biyan, YNSA Nose Point, Wrist Point 1.

Explanation

- **KI-3**, **KI-6**, **CV-4**, **CV-6**, **GV-4** and **BL-23** nourish and tonify the Kidney (for their different actions see Table 1.7.5).
  - Use moxa in the case of Kidney-Yang and Kidney-Jing deficiency.
- **ST-40** transforms Phlegm.
- **LI-20**, **BL-2**, **ST-2**, **ST-3**, **GB-14**, **GV-23**, Yintang, Yuyao, Taiyang, Bitong and Biyan benefit the nose and/or sinuses (congestion, discharge, pain, anosmia, sneezing).
  - Choose local points depending on the affected zones (see Tables 1.7.3 and 1.7.4).
- YNSA Nose Point or Wrist Point 1 is a good addition when the nose is hard to open.

Clinical Notes

- In the case of severe Kidney-Jing deficiency someone will *not* be fit to dive by any means. Clinical signs and symptoms like poor memory, forgetfulness and loose teeth are big risks for diving accidents (e.g. healthy denture is needed to keep the regulator well in the mouth).

Table 1.7.5 Different acupuncture points and the affected parts of the Kidney

Acupuncture points	Affected part
KI-1 Yongquan	Kidney-Yin
KI-3 Taixi	Kidney-Yin, Kidney-Yang
KI-6 Zhaohai	Kidney-Yin
CV-4 Guanyuan	Kidney-Yin, Kidney-Yang, Kidney-Jing
CV-6 Qihai	Kidney-Yang
GV-4 Mingmen	Especially Kidney-Yang; Kidney-Jing
BL-23 Shenshu	Kidney-Yin, Kidney-Yang, Kidney-Jing

4 Liver-Qi Stagnation Resulting in Liver and Gall Bladder-Fire

This pattern is often caused by chronic stress and emotional disturbances/restrictions (especially anger). Due to Liver-Qi stagnation Jin Ye congeal into Phlegm in the nose and sinuses. Prolonged Liver-Qi stagnation can end up in Liver and Gall Bladder-Fire, even with dryness of the mucosa as a result.

People with Liver-Qi stagnation feel better and are more productive when they move (like walking, cycling, swimming etc.) and express their emotions as this promotes the circulation of Liver-Qi.

● Clinical Signs and Symptoms

- Thick sticky yellow or green nasal discharge, purulent and smelling; or nasal congestion
- Inflamed swollen membranes (can become dry in the case of Liver and Gall Bladder-Fire)
- Anosmia
- Intense headache (frontal, temporal, or distension of the head)
- Maxillary pain
- Dizziness
- Tinnitus
- Red face, red/burning eyes
- Fever
- Bitter taste in the mouth, dry mouth, thirst
- Constipation or dry stools, pellet-shaped stools
- Insomnia or dream-disturbed sleep
- In general: feeling easily irritated or frustrated
- Pain or stiffness in the flanks.

Pulse: Wiry (*Xian*), Full (*Shi*) and Rapid (*Shuo*).

Tongue: Red with a yellow coating.

● Treatment Principle

– Spread Liver-Qi.

– Clear Liver and Gall Bladder-Fire.

– Transform Phlegm.

– Open the nose and sinuses.

● Acupuncture Points (select from)
LI-4 Hegu, **LIV-3** Taichong, **PC-6** Neiguan, **LIV-2** Xingjian, **GB-43** Xiaxi, **GB-39** Xuanzong, **LIV-8** Ququan, **ST-40** Fenglong, **LI-20** Yingxiang,

BL-2 Zanzhu, **ST-2** Sibai, **ST-3** Juliao, **GB-14** Yangbai, **GV-23** Shangxing, **M-HN-3** Yintang, **M-HN-6** Yuyao, **M-HN-9** Taiyang, **M-HN-14** Bitong, **(EX)** Biyan, YNSA Nose Point, Wrist Point 1.

- Explanation

  - **LI-4–LIV-3** combination and **PC-6** spread Liver-Qi.
  - **LIV-2**, **GB-43** and **GB-39** clear Liver and/or Gall Bladder-Fire.
  - **LIV-8** nourishes Liver-Yin and Liver-Xue to benefit dry mucosa (in the case of long-term Liver and Gall Bladder-Fire).
  - **ST-40** transforms Phlegm.
  - **LI-20**, **BL-2**, **ST-2**, **ST-3**, **GB-14**, **GV-23**, Yintang, Yuyao, Taiyang, Bitong and Biyan benefit the nose and sinuses (congestion, discharge, pain, anosmia, sneezing).
    - Choose local points depending on the affected zones (see Tables 1.3 and 1.4).
  - YNSA Nose Point or Wrist Point 1 is a good addition when the nose is hard to open.

- Clinical Notes

  - **LI-4–LIV-3** combination, also called the *Four Gates*, strongly promotes the free flow of Qi and Xue in the whole body and calms the Shen (Spirit). The Four Gates are Yuan Xue (Source Points) and this point combination works very well to treat Liver-Qi stagnation (stress, anger, frustration, depression). **LI-4** harmonizes the ascending and descending of Qi (which subdues Liver-Qi[87]). **LIV-3** is the most important point to spread Liver-Qi (which in turn provides a free flow of Qi in general).
  - **(EX)** Biyan opens the nose and is especially effective in the case of dryness of the mucosa due to long-term Liver-Qi stagnation/Liver and Gall Bladder-Fire.

- Food

Earl Grey tea helps to support relaxing the Liver. Fresh mint tea cools the Liver.

---

87 Maciocia, G., *The Foundations of Chinese Medicine: A Comprehensive Text*, third edition, Elsevier, Amsterdam, 2015.

- Lifestyle

Reduce stress by:

- relaxation
- meditation
- sports.

Advice for the Diver

- Don't dive while you have rhinosinusitis because clearing the ears and/or sinuses will not be possible (or will be insufficient) and there is a big risk of barotrauma.

- Avoid cold, hot and/or dry air in the face, such as air conditioning (home, office, plane), and in wintertime protect your forehead, neck and ears against cold and wind. Also protect yourself well when flying long-distance (fleece, shawl, blanket).

1.8 ALLERGIC RHINITIS AND NON-ALLERGIC RHINITIS
过敏性鼻炎

Western Medicine

Definition and Aetiology

Allergic rhinitis is an excessive immune response to foreign substances (inhalant allergens); histamine (among other things) is released in the nose under the influence of the binding of allergens to Immunoglobin (IgE) antibodies on mast cells. As a result, the permeability of the blood vessels in the nose increases and the nerve endings present in the nose are stimulated, resulting in hypersecretion, itching and sneezing.[88] Allergic rhinitis can be caused by dust mites, mould and pet dander (in all seasons; *perennial rhinitis*) or by pollen (seasonally; hay fever).

The medical history is very important when diagnosing allergic rhinitis. *If there isn't sneezing and itching it isn't an allergic rhinopathy!* If one parent has allergic rhinopathy the chance of the child being allergic is 40 per cent, and if both parents have allergic rhinopathy the chance of the child being allergic is 70 per cent. Skin tests are very reliable.

---

[88] NHG Standaard Allergische en niet-allergische rhinitis (Eerste herziening) Sachs, A.P.E., Berger, M.Y., Lucassen, P.L.B.J., Van der Wal, J., Van Balen, J.A.M., Verduijn, M.M., 'Huisarts Wet', (2006) 49, 5, 254–65.

Diagnosis

The clinical signs and symptoms of rhinitis are:

- nasal congestion or watery nasal discharge
- sneezing
- itching nose, throat, eyes
- watery eyes
- anosmia
- headache
- poor concentration
- sleepiness
- tiredness.

Non-allergic rhinitis (idiopathic or vasomotor rhinitis) is the hyperreactive reaction of the mucosa not caused by inhalant allergens but as a result of non-specific, non-immunological stimuli such as:

- compressed air
- temperature changes
- air conditioning
- humidity
- smoking
- alcohol
- medication (e.g. overuse of decongestant nasal spray (*rhinitis medicamentosa* or *rebound rhinitis*), NSAIDs such as ibuprofen and naproxen, oral contraceptives, beta-blockers)
- odours (paint, perfume, latex, cooking)
- tiredness
- stress
- physical exertion (e.g. repetitive dives)
- disturbed day/night transition.

Polyps are an expression of hyperreactivity of the mucosa.

BOX 1.8.1 ALLERGY AND HYPERREACTIVITY
If you are allergic you also are hyperreactive but if you are hyperreactive you aren't necessarily allergic. When you are infectious you are hyperreactive as well but not allergic.

Treatment

- Nasal and/or oral antihistamines (tablets side-effects: drowsiness, dry mouth): *only prescribed in the case of allergic rhinitis.*
- Nasal (preferred) or oral corticosteroids.
- Pseudoephedrine (e.g. Sudafed®) (side-effects: restlessness, stomach complaints, vomiting, dizziness, breathing problems, palpitations, hallucinations).
- Immunotherapy (in the case of allergic rhinitis): it's scientifically proven that immunotherapy affects the natural course of the condition, especially when there is mono-allergy; it's less effective when there is poly-allergy.

Clinical Notes

- It's important *not* to use *sedating* antihistamines when diving because drowsiness is one of the side-effects and the diver has to stay alert. Sedating antihistamines might provoke nitrogen narcosis whereby the sedating effect increases. *Non-sedating* antihistamines are *less* sedating but still can cause sedation. Aerius®, containing desloratadine, has few side-effects.[89]

Chinese Medicine
Definition and Aetiology

Allergic rhinitis (*Bi Qiu* or Snivelling Nose) implies that pathogenic Qi is invading the nose and irritating the mucosa if the Wei Qi is not strong enough or when the pathogen is very strong. When the mucous membranes are irritated they are more sensitive to other stimuli.

Allergic rhinitis is divided into:

- seasonal rhinitis: hay fever (trees, grasses)

---

[89] Meeuwis, C., Lecture: 'ENT medication and diving', Stichting Duik Research, Amsterdam, 2016.

- perennial rhinitis: rhinitis during the whole year (like an allergy for dogs and/or cats, dust mites).

For seasonal rhinitis, you should treat the root of the disorder, building up energy and improving immunity, out of season! In the season itself, you treat if complaints show up and a maintenance treatment of one time per four weeks is recommended to support the energy level.

Pattern Differentiation
1 Wind-Cold
An acute invasion of Wind-Cold attacks the nose and constricts the movement of Lung-Qi, thereby causing Jin Ye to stagnate and accumulate, and irritates the mucous membranes.

● Clinical Signs and Symptoms
- Sneezing
- Itchy nose
- Thin white or watery discharge (runny nose) or congestion
- Anosmia
- Itching, irritated and watery eyes
- Pale face
- Frontal headache or maxillary pain.

Pulse: Floating (*Fu*) and Tight (*Jin*).

Tongue: Normal (in the initial stage) or with a thin white coating.

● Treatment Principle
- Clear Wind-Cold.
- Promote the descending and diffusing of Lung-Qi.
- Open the nose.

● Acupuncture Points (select from)
LI-4 Hegu, **TB-5** Waiguan, **LU-7** Lieque, **BL-12** Fengmen, **BL-13** Feishu, **LI-20** Yingxiang, **M-HN-3** Yintang, **M-HN-14** Bitong, **(EX)** Biyan, YNSA Nose Point, **BL-2** Zanzhu, **M-HN-6** Yuyao, Ear Point: Allergy Point, **GB-20** Fengchi, **SP-6** Sanyinjiao, **ST-36** Zusanli.

Explanation

- **LI-4**, **LU-7** and **TB-5** expel Wind-Cold and release the exterior.
- **LU-7**, **BL-12** and **BL-13** promote the descending and diffusing of Lung-Qi (cough). Use **BL-12** in the early stage of the condition and **BL-13** in recurring pathology.
- **LI-20**, Yintang, Bitong and Biyan expel Wind and open the nose (congestion, discharge, sneezing, nasal itching, anosmia). **LI-20** and Bitong can be used for nasal polyps.
- YNSA Nose Point is a good addition when the nose is hard to open.
- **BL-2** expels Wind, benefits the eyes and nose.
- Yuyao benefits the eyes (lacrimation, itching, allergic conjunctivitis) and frontal headache.
- Ear Point: Allergy Point benefits allergies in general. Use a semi-permanent auricular needle.
- **GB-20** eliminates Wind from the head. Use in the case of blocked ears, a stiff neck or headache.
- **SP-6** and **ST-36** support general tonification and immunity.

2 Wind-Heat

Wind-Cold can turn into Wind-Heat or there might be an invasion of Wind-Heat that dries and damages Jin Ye, blocks the movement of Lung-Qi, and irritates the mucous membranes.

Clinical Signs and Symptoms

- Sneezing
- Itching of the nose or throat, sore throat
- Thick or yellow nasal discharge or congestion
- Anosmia
- Red, irritated, itching eyes
- Thirst
- Frontal headache or maxillary pain.

Pulse: Floating (*Fu*) and Rapid (*Shuo*).

Tongue: Normal (in the initial stage) or with a red front and thin yellow coating.

- Treatment Principle
    - Clear Wind-Heat.
    - Promote the descending and diffusing of Lung-Qi.
    - Open the nose.

- Acupuncture Points (select from)
  LI-4 Hegu, **LI-11** Quchi, **TB-5** Waiguan, **LU-5** Chize, **LU-10** Yuji, **LU-7** Lieque, **BL-12** Fengmen, **BL-13** Feishu, **GB-20** Fengchi, **LI-20** Yingxiang, **M-HN-3** Yintang, **M-HN-14** Bitong, **(EX)** Biyan, YNSA Nose Point, **BL-2** Zanzhu, **M-HN-6** Yuyao, Ear Point: Allergy Point, **SP-6** Sanyinjiao, **ST-36** Zusanli.

- Explanation
    - **LI-4**, **LI-11** and **TB-5** expel Wind-Heat and release the exterior.
    - **LU-5** (cough) and **LU-10** (no voice) clear Heat from the Lung.
    - **LU-7**, **BL-12** and **BL-13** promote the descending and diffusing of Lung-Qi.
    - **GB-20** eliminates Wind from the head. Use in the case of headache.
    - **LI-20**, Yintang, Bitong and Biyan expel Wind and open the nose. **LI-20** and Bitong can be used in case of nasal polyps.
    - YNSA Nose Point is a good addition when the nose is hard to open.
    - **BL-2** expels Wind, benefits the eyes and nose.
    - Yuyao benefits the eyes (lacrimation, itching, redness, allergic conjunctivitis) and frontal headache.
    - Ear Point: Allergy Point, benefits allergies in general. Use a semi-permanent auricular needle.
    - **SP-6** and **ST-36** support general tonification and immunity.

The Underlying Deficiency: Pattern Differentiation and Treatment

1 Lung-Qi Deficiency
Rhinitis based on deficiency of Lung-Qi is seen when there is a constitutional weakness of the Lung, prolonged sadness and grief, bad posture (sitting hunched causing superficial breathing), excessive talking, smoking and chronic or repetitive nose and/or sinus disorders.

EAR, NOSE AND THROAT DISORDERS

● Clinical Signs and Symptoms
- Clear watery discharge or nasal congestion
- Sneezing
- Itching nose
- Anosmia
- Shortness of breath
- Weak voice
- Dislike of talking
- Pale face
- Spontaneous sweating
- Cold wind/air increases the symptoms
- Frequent colds.

Pulse: Deficient (*Xu*) or Weak (*Ruo*).

Tongue: Pale with a thin white coating.

● Treatment Principle
– Tonify Lung-Qi.
– Transform Phlegm.
– Open the nose and benefit the eyes.

● Acupuncture Points (select from)
LU-7 Lieque, **LU-9** Taiyuan, **BL-13** Feishu, **ST-40** Fenglong, **LI-20** Yingxiang, **M-HN-3** Yintang, **M-HN-14** Bitong, **(EX)** Biyan, YNSA Nose Point, **BL-2** Zanzhu, **M-HN-6** Yuyao, Ear Point: Allergy Point, **SP-6** Sanyinjiao, **ST-36** Zusanli.

● Explanation
- **LU-7**, **LU-9** and **BL-13** tonify Lung-Qi.
- **ST-40** transforms Phlegm.
- **LI-20**, Yintang, Bitong and Biyan open the nose. **LI-20** and Bitong can be used in the case of nasal polyps.
- YNSA Nose Point is a good addition when the nose is hard to open.

- **BL-2** benefits the eyes and nose.
- Yuyao benefits the eyes (lacrimation, itching, allergic conjunctivitis).
- Ear Point: Allergy Point benefits allergies in general. Use a semi-permanent auricular needle.
- **SP-6** and **ST-36** support general tonification and immunity.

2 Spleen-Qi Deficiency

Deficiency of the Spleen is often caused by obsessive thinking, irregular meals, bad diet (too much sugar, cold foods) and the regular use of antibiotics.

This category based on Spleen-Qi deficiency includes hyperreactivity to fumes and cigarette smoke.[90]

● Clinical Signs and Symptoms

- Thin watery or sticky white discharge or nasal congestion
- Pale and swollen mucosa
- Sneezing
- Itching nose
- Anosmia
- Tiredness especially in the morning
- Heavy-feeling head and woolly-headed
- Heavy limbs
- Poor appetite
- Distension (abdomen, epigastrium)
- Borborygmus
- Loose stools
- Aversion to cold.

Pulse: Deficient (*Xu*) or Weak (*Ruo*).
In case of Damp/Phlegm due to weak Spleen-Qi the pulse will be Slippery (*Hua*).

Tongue: Pale, swollen and tooth marks, with a white coating.

----

90 Maclean, W. and Lyttleton, J., *Clinical Handbook of Internal Medicine*, Volume 1, fifth printing, University of Western Sydney, Sydney, 2008.

- Treatment Principle
    - Tonify Spleen-Qi.
    - Transform Dampness/Phlegm.
    - Open the nose and benefit the eyes.

- Acupuncture Points (select from)
SP-6 Sanyinjiao, **SP-4** Gongsun, **SP-3** Taibai, **BL-20** Pishu, **SP-9** Yinlingquan, **CV-12** Zhongwan, **ST-36** Zusanli, **ST-40** Fenglong, **LI-20** Yingxiang, **M-HN-3** Yintang, **M-HN-14** Bitong, **(EX)** Biyan, YNSA Nose Point, **BL-2** Zanzhu, **M-HN-6** Yuyao, Ear Point: Allergy Point.

- Explanation

    - **SP-6**, **SP-4**, **SP-3** and **BL-20** tonify Spleen-Qi and resolve Dampness. **SP-6** supports general tonification and immunity as well.

    - **SP-9** and **CV-12** resolve Dampness.

    - **ST-36** fortifies the Spleen, resolves Dampness and Phlegm, supports general tonification and immunity.

    - **ST-40** transforms Phlegm.

    - **LI-20**, Yintang, Bitong and Biyan open the nose. **LI-20** and Bitong can be used in the case of nasal polyps.

    - YNSA Nose Point is a good addition when the nose is hard to open.

    - **BL-2** benefits the eyes and nose.

    - Yuyao benefits the eyes.

    - Ear Point: Allergy Point, benefits allergies in general. Use a semi-permanent auricular needle.

CASE STUDY 1.8.1 HYPERREACTIVITY MUCOSA

A young budding diver (14 years, male) exercising for the first diving licence (*Open Water*) had to stop the diving lessons because of equalization problems (right ear) due to a completely blocked nose.

Medical History
The boy visited a diving medicine physician specializing in ENT disorders and was advised to stop diving because it was not possible for him to clear his right ear at all (including above the water surface). Under water the equalizing problem

started at just 1 metre depth! Research from the ENT doctor concluded that he had a narrow Eustachian tube without the presence of an allergy. He had had problems with inflammations of the ear from childhood; he had grommets in the tympanic membranes several times and had a common cold a couple of times per year (the last time being two months before the treatment). Antibiotics were used frequently. The budding diver arrived at my practice looking extremely tired, and his nose was noticeably blocked (specifically swollen membranes, mucus less pronounced). He had a lack of Shen (no gloss at the eyes), problems getting up in the morning, concentration problems at school and, regarding diet, was drinking a lot of fizzy drinks daily.

Chinese Medicine Diagnosis
Lung-Qi, Spleen-Qi and Kidney-Yin deficiency.

Treatment

- Tonify the Lung-Qi and Spleen-Qi: **LU-7** Lieque, **LU-9** Taiyuan, **SP-3** Taibai, **SP-4** Gongsun and **SP-6** Sanyinjiao.

- Nourish Kidney-Yin: **KI-3** Taixi, **KI-6** Zhaohai, **CV-4** Guanyuan and **CV-6** Qihai.

- Support general health: **ST-36** Zusanli.

- Transform Phlegm: **ST-40** Fenglong.

- Open the nose: **M-HN-3** Yintang, **(EX)** Biyan, **LI-20** Yingxiang, **LI-4** Hegu and Allergy Point both ears.

Result
During the first treatment it was obvious the nose opened and the diver felt more air coming through the nostrils. After four treatments the diver was able to clear both ears directly after the treatment (out of water). After eight treatments the diver went to the course again. Ear-clearing under water went well and he passed the diving exam. His energy level improved a lot, concentration at school was much better and he became a more active and happy person.

CASE STUDY 1.8.2 REVERSE BLOCK

Diver, 40 years old, male, instructor on live-a-boards (where participants stay on a boat for several days) in Egypt.

Medical History
Complaints in the frontal sinuses while ascending. Going through horrible pain to get back to the water surface. He felt stressed not being able to work. Surgery (restoring the natural ostium; the diver came to the Netherlands especially for this surgery), medication (antibiotics), anti-inflammatory nose drops (Flixonase, which contains corticosteroids). No result. His overall resistance was weak due to long working days and few free days in between the groups of divers on the live-a-boards.

Chinese Medicine Diagnosis
Lung-Qi and Spleen-Qi deficiency; Phlegm; Liver-Qi stagnation.

Treatment
- Tonify Lung-Qi and Spleen-Qi: **LU-7** Lieque, **LU-9** Taiyuan, **SP-4** Gongsun, **SP-6** Sanyinjiao and **ST-36** Zusanli.
- Transform Phlegm: **ST-40** Fenglong.
- Open the nose and frontal sinuses: **M-HN-3** Yintang, **M-HN-6** Yuyao, **(EX)** Biyan, **LI-20** Yingxiang and **LI-4** Hegu.
- Promote the smooth flow of Liver-Qi: **LI-4** Hegu, **LIV-3** Taichong and **PC-6** Neiguan.

Result
Totally free from complaints after six treatments. The diver returned to the Red Sea to work as an instructor again. Six months after finishing the acupuncture sessions he emailed me to tell me that ascending in the water still went without any problems.

3 Kidney Deficiency
In hereditary allergic rhinitis there is usually deficiency of the Kidney (or Lung) and the allergy presents at an early age. Kidney deficiency also occurs due to chronic illness, overwork, excessive sexual activity (which depletes Kidney-Jing especially), loss of Jin Ye and/or Xue (Kidney-Yin deficiency), emotional strain (fear) and ageing.

● Clinical Signs and Symptoms
- Nasal congestion (dry, atrophic, scabbed mucosa in the case of Yin deficiency) or watery discharge in the case of Yang deficiency (worse in morning and evening)

- Itching nose
- Sneezing
- Anosmia.

● Kidney-Yin Deficiency: Clinical Signs and Symptoms
- Five-palm Heat
- Insomnia
- Tinnitus
- Dizziness
- Weakness and pain in the lower back.

Pulse: Thready (*Xi*) and Rapid (*Shuo*).

Tongue: Red and dry with little or no coating.

● Kidney-Yang Deficiency: Clinical Signs and Symptoms
- Aversion to cold
- Cold feeling in the lower back and knees
- Cold limbs
- Low libido, infertility
- Tiredness
- Lethargy, no motivation
- Pale face
- Frequent urination in the night with copious clear urine
- Pale urine.

Pulse: Deep (*Chen*), Thready (*Xi*) and Slow (*Chi*).

Tongue: Pale and swollen with a white coating.

● Kidney-Jing Deficiency: Clinical Signs and Symptoms
- Sore and weak lower back and knees
- Tinnitus, deafness
- Blurred vision

- Infertility, low libido
- Falling or (premature) greying hair
- Loose teeth
- Bone problems (development, softening)
- Forgetfulness and poor memory.

There may be no specific Hot or Cold signs if Kidney-Yin and Kidney-Yang are equally weak.

Pulse: Deep (*Chen*), Thready (*Xi*) and Weak (*Ruo*).

Tongue: Variable depending on whether there is more Yin or Yang deficiency.

● Treatment Principle

- Nourish and tonify Kidney-Yin, Kidney-Yang and/or Kidney-Jing.
- Open the nose.
- Transform Phlegm.

● Acupuncture Points (select from)

KI-3 Taixi, **KI-6** Zhaohai, **CV-4** Guanyuan, **CV-6** Qihai, **GV-4** Mingmen, **BL-23** Shenshu, **ST-40** Fenglong, **LI-20** Yingxiang, **M-HN-3** Yintang, **M-HN-14** Bitong, **(EX)** Biyan, YNSA Nose Point, **BL-2** Zanzhu, **M-HN-6** Yuyao, Ear Point: Allergy Point.

● Explanation

- **KI-3**, **KI-6**, **CV-4**, **CV-6**, **GV-4** and **BL-23** nourish and tonify the Kidney (for their different actions see Table 1.7.5).
  - Use moxa in the case of Kidney-Yang and Kidney-Jing deficiency.
- **ST-40** transforms Phlegm.
- **LI-20**, Yintang, Bitong and Biyan open the nose. **LI-20** and Bitong can be used in the case of nasal polyps.
- YNSA Nose Point is a good addition when the nose is hard to open.
- **BL-2** benefits the eyes and nose.
- Yuyao benefits the eyes.
- Ear Point: Allergy Point benefits allergies in general. Use a semi-permanent auricular needle.

⬇ Advice for the Diver

- Never dive when you have an acute nasal allergy (e.g. hay fever) because there is a big risk that you won't be able to clear the ears.

- Don't dive if you have taken antihistamines that make you sleepy. During diving you have to act and react accurately and be alert the whole time.

- Don't smoke! Nicotine causes phlegm and irritates the mucous membranes in the nose, sinuses and lungs. Acupuncture can help to stop smoking addiction.

- Eat healthy food (a diet with lots of fat and sugar produces phlegm).

- Prevent the influence of air-conditioning (airplane, hotel room, restaurant) and big differences in temperature, which make the mucosa in the nose, sinuses and Eustachian tube dry and sensitive.

- When you have sensitive mucous membranes in the nose and sinuses it's better to make one dive per day so there is enough recovery time for the mucosa.

- Take enough time to acclimatize after arriving at your diving destination. One day's rest is recommended after a long flight with little sleep, air conditioning, dehydration of the body and when having jet lag due to different time zones. A good recovery from the travel can reduce the risk of irritation of the mucosa in the nose and sinuses and decompression illness.

1.9 OTITIS
耳炎

Otitis externa, media and interna are contraindications for diving (temporary dive ban) because clearing the ears can't be done properly. In otitis media there is no open air passage to the Eustachian tube, which implies a big risk of rupture of the tympanic membrane and damaging the ossicles and the labyrinth, with loss of hearing or tinnitus as a result.

Otitis externa is one of the most seen disorders experienced by divers. It occurs frequently because bacteria from the oceans, lakes and swimming pools easily enter the external acoustic meatus, which can lead to infection and inflammation. The inflammation of the skin can block the external acoustic meatus, creating a vacuum whereby equalization is not possible and a perforation of the tympanic membrane can occur.

Hygiene and an open Eustachian tube are of indisputable importance in preventing ear disorders. Never put your finger in your ear after diving in the sea or ocean! This will damage the skin, which has become sensitive due to the salty sea water. The bacteria and salt crystals can enter the skin directly, the bacteria can multiply quickly – especially when it's warm and humid – and the chance is very high that you will have an otitis externa the next day.

People with seborrheic eczema and psoriasis are at higher risk of getting otitis externa after swimming or diving in warm polluted water,[91] because of the skin flakes.

Western Medicine
Definition and Aetiology

Otitis is an inflammation in the external, middle or inner ear due to an infection, eczema, psoriasis, allergy, diabetes or an auto-immune disease. An infection implies there is contamination by bacteria, fungi or viruses, which enter the ear, nose or mouth.

General signs of an inflammation are pain, heat, swelling, redness and loss of function.

BOX 1.9.1 THE OCCURRENCE OF OTITIS CAUSED BY BACTERIA, VIRUSES AND FUNGI

Contamination ➔ Infection ➔ Inflammation

Otitis Externa (e.g. Swimmer's Ear)

Otitis Externa is an inflammation of the skin in the external acoustic meatus and is often caused by the bacteria Pseudomonas aeruginosa and Staphylococcus aureus.

Clinical Signs and Symptoms

- Ear pain
- Itching in the ear
- Skin flakes
- Conductive hearing loss
- Ear discharge
- Slight fever

---

91 Brandt Corstius, J.J., Dermout, S.M. and Feenstra, L., *Duikgeneeskunde, Theorie en Praktijk*, tweede druk, Elsevier, Amsterdam, 2007.

- Sometimes tinnitus
- Swelling of the skin (the external acoustic meatus can be blocked totally).

Otitis Media

Acute otitis media (AOM) is usually caused by Streptococcus pneumoniae, Haemophilus influenzae or Moraxella catarrhalis. It is also possible that there is liquid effusion in the middle ear *without* an infection (otitis media with effusion: OME). OME might occur when the acute ear inflammation is resolved or if the Eustachian tube is partly blocked which allows fluid to build up (and this situation can result in an infection).

Clinical Signs and Symptoms

- Ear pain (often with thumping character)
- Conductive hearing loss
- Ear discharge (purulent or liquid effusion)
- There might be perforation of the tympanic membrane due to the high pressure of the purulent discharge
- Fever
- Pulsating tinnitus
- Sometimes dizziness.

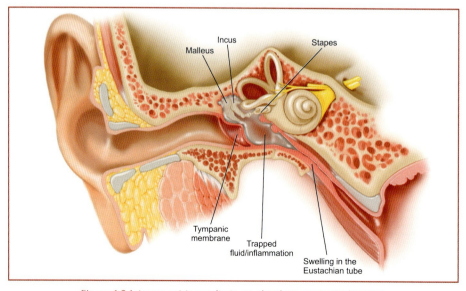

Figure 1.9.1 Acute otitis media is an absolute contraindication for diving because it will be impossible to clear the affected ear

Otitis Interna (Labyrinthitis)

Otitis interna often occurs due to a virus (e.g. after a common cold or flu), and sometimes after a bacterial middle ear infection or meningitis.

Clinical Signs and Symptoms

- Ear pain
- Feeling of pressure in the ear
- Acute dizziness
- Loss of balance
- Nausea
- Vomiting
- Tinnitus
- Hearing loss
- Fever.

Diagnosis

Otoscopy by an ENT doctor or general physician.

Treatment

- Decongestion: nose drops (xylometazoline, for example Otrivin®).
- Painkillers.
- Antibiotics (oral and/or topical).
- Acid drops in the case of an otitis externa (0.2 ml acetic acid in 10 ml isopropyl alcohol, prepared by a pharmacy).[92]
- In the early stages otitis externa can be treated with iodine injected by an ENT physician in the external acoustic meatus.

---

92 Brandt Corstius, J.J., Dermout, S.M. and Feenstra, L., *Duikgeneeskunde, Theorie en Praktijk*, tweede druk, Elsevier, Amsterdam, 2007.

Chinese Medicine
Definition and Aetiology

An external pathogenic Qi can enter the nose or ear and attack the energy system when the Wei Qi is not strong enough, when the pathogen is very strong or when the body is not protected well. Otitis can be a result of a badly healed acute common cold or flu. Internal energetic disbalance (fullness, emptiness) can likewise lead to ear inflammations.

Otitis externa is caused by external factors but can be triggered internally, for example by skin flakes due to eczema. Otitis media and interna are caused by external factors (Wind-Heat, virus, bacteria) and internal factors (e.g. an allergy or auto-immune disease). This signifies that there are underlying deficiencies or other energetic disbalances (Liver, Gall Bladder, Kidney), which affect the onset of the inflammation.

Acupuncture treatment can improve the total energy level of a person and the local condition in the Eustachian tube and middle ear as well as relieving pain and pressure in the ear.

In general acupuncture can prevent a middle ear infection when the focus is to transform Dampness and/or Phlegm and to diminish swelling of the mucosa in the Eustachian tube. This way the middle ear can be ventilated through the Eustachian tube, which prevents a breeding ground for micro-organisms.

Pattern Differentiation
1 Damp-Heat Liver-Gall Bladder

The most common type seen with inflammations in the ear is the excess type. There is Damp-Heat in the Liver-Gall Bladder, often accompanied with a diet with too much fat and hot food/drinks.

- Clinical Signs and Symptoms

    - Yellow purulent ear discharge with foul smell
    - Ear pain
    - Hearing loss
    - Tinnitus
    - Bitter taste in the mouth
    - Headache, heavy head
    - Fever
    - Red eyes

- Constipation or dry stools
- Poor appetite
- Nausea, vomiting
- Chest or hypochondriac distension
- Swelling or itching of the genitals.

Pulse: Slippery (*Hua*), Wiry (*Xian*) and Rapid (*Shuo*).

Tongue: Red with a sticky yellow coating.

● Treatment Principle

– Clear Damp-Heat from the Liver-Gall Bladder.
– Open the ears.

● Acupuncture Points (select from)

GB-34 Yanglingquan, **GB-43** Xiaxi, **GB-42** Diwuhui, **LIV-2** Xingjian, **LIV-3** Taichong, **TB-3** Zhongzhu, **SP-9** Yinlingquan, **CV-12** Zhongwan, **TB-21** Ermen, **SI-19** Tinggong, **GB-2** Tinghui, **TB-17** Yifeng, **ST-7** Xiaguan, YNSA Ear Point, Wrist Point 4.

● Explanation

- **GB-34** and **GB-43** clear Damp-Heat from the Liver-Gall Bladder (differentiation: organ **GB-34** and channel **GB-43**).
- **GB-42** clears Heat from the Gall Bladder, improves hearing acuity.
- **LIV-2** and **LIV-3** clear Liver-Fire.
- **TB-3** clears Heat of the head and is a strong working distal point in ear disorders like otitis, tinnitus and deafness.
- **SP-9** and **CV-12** to support transforming Dampness in general.
- **TB-21**, **SI-19**, **GB-2** and **TB-17** clear Heat, benefit the ears and improve hearing acuity.
- **ST-7** clears Heat from the ears.
- YNSA Ear Point, Wrist Point 4 benefit the ears.

DIVING MEDICAL ACUPUNCTURE

● Clinical Notes

- **TB-3** is useful in the case of obstruction of the ear due to Phlegm-Damp or Phlegm-Heat.[93] According to Deadman, Al-Khafaji and Baker you can massage this point 'during or following flying' when having blocked ears combined with equalization.[94] Clearing techniques that can be performed easily are swallowing, bringing the mandible forward and downwards, or the Valsalva manoeuvre. The latter one can be performed *with caution*. Equalizing too forcefully means that the pressure change may be too extreme and you can damage the round or oval window of the inner ear. I would advise using the mandible movement only a couple of times otherwise it may irritate the TMJ.

- In the case of a *blocked ear* (pressure and associated hearing loss) after having had otitis media I experience very good results when needling **SI-19** to open the Eustachian tube. Most of the time two treatments are sufficient to get rid of the ear pressure and hearing loss.

> ### BOX 1.9.2 EAR POINTS AND EAR STRUCTURES
> The ear points **TB-21** Ermen, **SI-19** Tinggong, **GB-2** Tinghui and **TB-17** Yifeng open the *ear orifices* and affect the external, middle and inner ear and the Eustachian tube.

> ### BOX 1.9.3 NEEDLING TECHNIQUE: SI-19 AND GB-2
> When needling **SI-19** and **GB-2** the mouth should be opened to create space for the needle in between the condyloid process of the mandible and the styloid process.

2 Liver-Yin and Kidney-Yin Deficiency
The deficiency type of ear inflammation concerns Liver-Yin and Kidney-Yin deficiency with Liver-Yang rising to the affected ear.

● Clinical Signs and Symptoms

- Clear thin discharge without foul smell (deficiency Heat)
- Ear pain
- Tinnitus

---

93 Deadman, P., Al-Khafaji, M. and Baker, K., *A Manual of Acupuncture*, Journal of Chinese Medicine Publications, Hove, 2015.
94 Deadman, P., Al-Khafaji, M. and Baker, K., *A Manual of Acupuncture*, Journal of Chinese Medicine Publications, Hove, 2015 (p.394).

- Hearing loss
- Headache
- Tiredness
- Night sweats
- Five-palm Heat
- Weak lower back/knees
- Insomnia
- Muscle weakness, cramps
- Dry eyes, blurred vision
- Brittle nails, dry hair and/or skin.

Pulse: Thready (*Xi*) and Rapid (*Shuo*).

Tongue: Red with little or no coating.

● Treatment Principle
  - Nourish Liver-Yin and Kidney-Yin.
  - Subdue Liver-Yang.
  - Open the ears.

● Acupuncture Points (select from)
LIV-3 Taichong, **LIV-8** Ququan, **BL-18** Ganshu, **KI-3** Taixi, **KI-6** Zhaohai, **BL-23** Shenshu, **LIV-2** Xingjian, **TB-3** Zhongzhu, **GB-20** Fengchi, **LI-11** Quchi, **TB-21** Ermen, **SI-19** Tinggong, **GB-2** Tinghui, **TB-17** Yifeng, YNSA Ear Point, Wrist Point 4.

● Explanation
- **LIV-3**, **LIV-8** and **BL-18** nourish Liver-Yin.
- **KI-3**, **KI-6** and **BL-23** nourish Kidney-Yin (nourishing the ears).
- **LIV-2**, **TB-3** and **GB-20** subdue Liver-Yang and benefit the ears.
- **LI-11** clears internal Heat. Add in case there is fever.
- **TB-21**, **SI-19**, **GB-2** and **TB-17** benefit the ears and improve hearing acuity.
- YNSA Ear Point and Wrist Point 4 benefit the ears.

3 External Type: Wind-Heat

The ear is attacked by an external invasion of Wind-Heat (think of driving with open windows in a jeep or pickup to a diving destination in desert countries located on the Red Sea, like Egypt, Jordan, Sudan and Saudi Arabia with strong and hot winds in summer).

● Clinical Signs and Symptoms

- Purulent or bloody exudate from the ear
- Distension/fullness in the ear
- Ear pain
- Headache
- Body ache
- Fever
- Thirst
- Aversion to wind.

Pulse: Floating (*Fu*) and Rapid (*Shuo*).

Tongue: Normal (in the initial stage) or with a thin white or yellow coating.

● Treatment Principle

- Clear Wind-Heat.
- Open the ears.

● Acupuncture Points (select from)

LI-4 Hegu, **LI-11** Quchi, **TB-5** Waiguan, **TB-3** Zhongzhu, **SI-3** Houxi, **GB-20** Fengchi, **TB-21** Ermen, **SI-19** Tinggong, **GB-2** Tinghui, **TB-17** Yifeng, **ST-7** Xiaguan, YNSA Ear Point, Wrist Point 4.

● Explanation

- **LI-4**, **LI-11** and **TB-5** expel Wind-Heat and release the exterior.
- **TB-3** and **SI-3** clear Wind-Heat. **TB-3** is a strong working distal point to benefit the ears. Add **SI-3** when there is a stiff neck or neck pain.
- **GB-20** eliminates Wind and is helpful in the case of blocked ears and headache.

EAR, NOSE AND THROAT DISORDERS

- **TB-21**, **SI-19**, **GB-2** and **TB-17** expel Wind from the ears, clear Heat, benefit the ears and improve hearing acuity.

- **ST-7** eliminates Wind, useful in the case of fullness of Yang in the ear,[95] and improves hearing acuity.

- YNSA Ear Point and Wrist Point 4 benefit the ears.

Table 1.9.1 Important acupuncture points to benefit the ears

Local points	Distal points	Special points/zones
TB-21 Ermen	**TB-3** Zhongzhu	Vertigo and Auditory Zone
SI-19 Tinggong	**TB-2** Yemen	YNSA Ear Point
GB-2 Tinghui	**GB-43** Xiaxi	Wrist Point 4
TB-17 Yifeng	**GB-42** Diwuhui	Ear Points: Inner Ear.C, Inner Ear.E
GB-20 Fengchi	**LIV-2** Xingjian	
	KI-3 Taixi	
	KI-1 Yongquan	

The *Vertigo and Auditory Zone* from Chinese Scalp Acupuncture has a length of 4 cm and is located 1.5 cm above the auricular apex, 2 cm ventral and 2 cm dorsal from the ear (see Figure 1.7.2). You must find the most tender point in this reflex zone and needle in the direction of the ear. You can treat the affected side or both sides. This zone is helpful in tinnitus, hearing impairment, dizziness and vertigo (a technique I learned at the China Beijing International Acupuncture Training Centre in 2004).

⬇ Advice for the Diver (and Any Other Watersporter) on How to Care for the Ears

- You mustn't dive (or swim/surf) when you have an ear inflammation! The ear must be treated carefully and after that examined by a doctor before going to dive again.

- Clean the ears with mineral water (when you are still on the diving boat or ashore) or shower water after every dive. Don't use a towel, handkerchief or cotton bud to dry the external ear canal because it might irritate the skin. Dry with a hair dryer instead.

---

95 Boermeester, W., *Tekstboek Acupunctuur, deel I, Punten*, Chinese Medicine Data, Kapellen, 1989.

- *Before* diving you can use drops of sunflower oil, olive oil or peanut oil (arachidis oleum)[96] to bring a protective layer on the skin of the external ear canal and tympanic membrane. If you want to use peanut oil be sure you have no peanut allergy! It is also possible to use *Earol Swim® Tea Tree Oil*, a formula that combines olive oil with tea tree oil, or *AudiolSWIM®*, which is 0.5 per cent tea tree oil 'per 10 ml medically filtered' olive oil. Tea tree oil is *Melaleuca alternifolia*, an essential oil native to Australia, which can work as an antiseptic, anti-inflammatory and antifungal.

- *After* diving use acid drops, which are prepared especially by the pharmacy (0.2 ml acetic acid in 10 ml isopropyl alcohol).[97] This acid will create an acidic environment in the external ear canal in which bacteria can't survive.

- Don't put a finger or anything else into your ears after diving! The finger will damage the skin, which has become sensitive from the salty sea water and you will push bacteria and salt crystals into the skin. This usually results in an external ear infection the day after the dive.

- Don't use headphones during a diving holiday. Headphones can damage the skin and make it prone to infection/inflammation.

BOX 1.9.4 SWIMMER'S EAR (A FORM OF OTITIS EXTERNA)

Excessive exposure to water and water retention in the external acoustic meatus can lead to otitis externa as bacteria can multiply quickly in a humid and warm surrounding. Less commonly, swimmer's ear can be caused by water contaminated with viruses or fungi. Water (especially salty sea water) that is retained in the external acoustic meatus softens the skin which can then easily be damaged by, for example, scratching, cleaning with cotton swabs or using headphones. Bacteria and salt crystals can enter the skin and cause infection followed by inflammation. The water of the oceans, seas, lakes and swimming pools contains lots of microbes. Swimmer's ear is seen a lot with watersporters but also can also happen if the ears are not cleaned and dried well after taking a bath or shower or being in the rain.

---

96 Brandt Corstius, J.J., Dermout, S.M. and Feenstra, L., *Duikgeneeskunde, Theorie en Praktijk*, tweede druk, Elsevier, Amsterdam, 2007.
97 Brandt Corstius, J.J., Dermout, S.M. and Feenstra, L., *Duikgeneeskunde, Theorie en Praktijk*, tweede druk, Elsevier, Amsterdam, 2007.

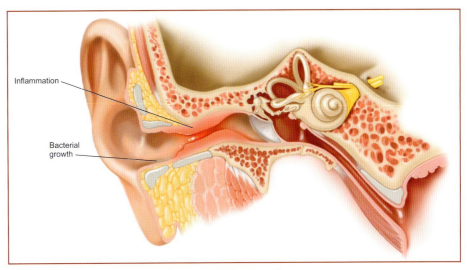

Figure 1.9.2 Swimmer's ear

1.10 SURFER'S EAR
冲浪耳

Surfers deal with the fact that they are in the overturning waves all the time, and the *water* and the *wind* hit the external acoustic meatus and tympanic membrane. The cold water impinges on the external acoustic meatus and irritates the skin and bone. This stimulates temporal bone growth and often leads to the formation of exostosis. The same thing can happen with swimmers and divers when they are frequently in cold water. The body protects against the cold water by creating an extra layer of bone around the external acoustic meatus. Surfer's ear develops in '80% of surfers' in cold wind and water conditions after 'ten years of water activity or 3,000 hours of surfing'.[98]

It is recommended that surfers and swimmers protect their ears with solid earplugs so the cold water cannot enter and damage the external acoustic meatus.

In wintertime and when surfing in cold wind and water conditions it's advisable to wear a neoprene hood to protect the skull. The cranium itself gets cold from the cold wind and water and surfer's ear can develop that way too.

In the Netherlands where I had surf lessons for a while – to understand more about specific medical problems experienced by surfers – the seawater is very cold. Even in summertime protection is needed.

---

98 Surfer Today, 'Surfer's Ear: Prevention and Protection', www.surfertoday.com/surfing/7720-surfers-ear-prevention-and-protection (accessed 10 August 2017).

DIVING MEDICAL ACUPUNCTURE

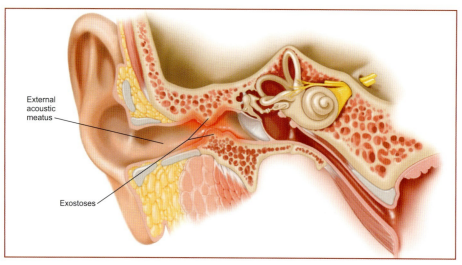

Figure 1.10.1 Surfer's ear with exostoses in the external acoustic meatus

> ### BOX 1.10.1 EARPLUGS
>
> For divers solid (*non-vented*) earplugs are strongly discouraged because under water they create a vacuum (under pressure) between the earplug and the tympanic membrane. This vacuum results in overpressure in the middle ear, which can lead to a rupture of the tympanic membrane while descending in the water.
>
> There are *vented* earplugs with a pressure valve that might support ear clearing by regulating a more gradual pressure change at the tympanic membrane, but there are risks of malfunction and removal.

A neoprene hood is advisable to protect the head from cooling when diving in cold water, when making deep dives where the water will be colder, or when diving frequently (e.g. a diving instructor and Divemaster).

When there are large exostoses obstructing the external acoustic meatus totally – or partially with swelling of the skin – and influencing the hearing capacity, the only solution is surgery (i.e. chiselling the exostosis). After surgery the ear needs rest for at least three weeks and a check by a physician before starting watersports again.

For surfer's ear acupuncture is not effective. Keeping the ears warm before and after surfing besides using earplugs and a neoprene hood are the best ways to prevent it.

1.11 PERFORATION OF THE TYMPANIC MEMBRANE
鼓膜穿孔

Western Medicine

Definition and Aetiology

Ignoring pressure on the tympanic membrane can result in a perforation (a traumatic deviation of the tympanic membrane, a hole or rupture, caused by under or overpressure). If this happens under water it is a very dangerous situation, which can lead to drowning. When the cold water enters the middle ear (through the perforation), the vestibular organ will be stimulated and caloric vertigo with disorientation, nausea and tinnitus can occur. If disoriented the diver may not be able to find his or her inflator/deflator and when the buddy is not alert the incident can have a fatal ending. The first thing the diver has to do in this situation is to put one finger in the external acoustic meatus by which the temperature in the ear will normalize and the symptoms will thus reduce.

The risk of a perforation emphasizes the importance of an open airway between the nose and middle ear, which is the first condition for clearing the ears well. As well as allowing air into the middle ear, the equalizing technique has to be done in a proper way and with sufficient frequency. As discussed before (see Section 1.4) there are different techniques from which the diver can choose the one that feels the best. Most divers clear by pinching the nose with the thumb and forefinger and breathing out through the nose (Valsalva manoeuvre) by which air will be brought to the middle ear whereby the position of the tympanic membrane will be neutralized.

Diagnosis
Otoscopy by an ENT doctor or general physician.

Clinical Signs and Symptoms

- Perforation
- Ear pain and pressure (relieved by the perforation)
- Discharge (fluids, blood)
- Hearing loss
- Tinnitus
- Caloric vertigo (stops when the ear has returned to normal temperature)
- Nausea, vomiting,

Treatment

Rest. Nose drops to be sure the Eustachian tube is open so there is no pressure on the tympanic membrane, by which it can heal. Usually it will take about six weeks before the tympanic membrane is cured. In the case of a large perforation surgery might be needed.

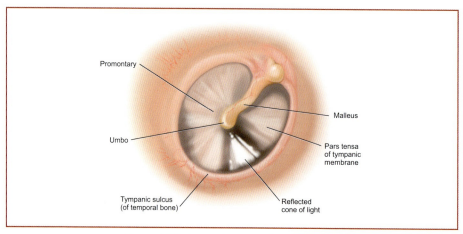

Figure 1.11.1a Normal tympanic membrane
Copyright © Terry Oleson

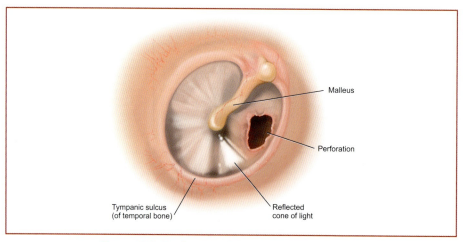

Figure 1.11.1b Perforation of the tympanic membrane
Copyright © Terry Oleson

Chinese Medicine

- Diagnosis

A perforation of the tympanic membrane only can be diagnosed objectively by means of otoscopy by an ENT doctor or general physician.

EAR, NOSE AND THROAT DISORDERS

● Clinical Signs and Symptoms
- Perforation
- Ear pain and pressure (relieved by the perforation)
- Discharge (fluids, blood)
- Hearing loss
- Tinnitus
- Caloric vertigo (stops when the ear has normal temperature again)
- Nausea, vomiting.

● Treatment
Same as the Western protocol: rest. Acupuncture and/or natural nose drops to be sure the nose and Eustachian tube are open so there is no pressure at the tympanic membrane, by which it can heal. Support any underlying energetic disbalance diagnosed by pulse, tongue and/or face.

● Treatment Principle
- Treat the underlying deficiency, fullness or stagnation.
- Open the nose, Eustachian tube and ears.

● Acupuncture Points (select from)
LI-4 Hegu, **LI-20** Yingxiang, **M-HN-3** Yintang, **(EX)** Biyan, **ST-40** Fenglong, **CV-12** Zhongwan, **TB-21** Ermen, **SI-19** Tinggong, **GB-2** Tinghui, **TB-17** Yifeng, **TB-3** Zhongzhu, YNSA Ear Point, Vertigo and Auditory Zone.

● Explanation
- **LI-4**, **LI-20**, Yintang and Biyan open the nose.
- **ST-40** and **CV-12** transform Phlegm.
- **TB-21**, **SI-19**, **GB-2**, **TB-17**, **TB-3**, YNSA Ear Point and the Vertigo and Auditory Zone benefit the ears and support the healing process of the tympanic membrane. **TB-21**, **SI-19**, **GB-2** and **TB-17** open the Eustachian tube from the middle ear side.

● Clinical Notes
- The acupuncture points that affect the nose open the Eustachian tube from the nasopharynx side.

⬇ Advice for the Diver

- When your eardrum ruptures under water and the cold water enters your ear you will have to put one finger in the external ear canal directly to protect the middle and inner ear. When no more cold water can penetrate, the temperature in the ear will increase and the dizziness will diminish. Of course you will have to terminate the dive and consult a physician.

- *After the perforation:* Prevent coughing, sneezing and squeezing as it can open the tympanic membrane during its healing process.

- *Caution:* Don't dive, swim, surf or fly for a minimum of six weeks and have a check-up with an ENT physician before diving again! You must be sure the eardrum is healed completely.

1.12 TINNITUS
耳鸣

Western Medicine
Definition and Aetiology

Tinnitus (ringing in the ears) is the perception of sound in the ear in the absence of a corresponding external stimulus, also called 'a phantom auditory perception'.[99] There is a differentiation between objective and subjective tinnitus. Objective tinnitus, which can be heard during examination by a physician (for example by stethoscopy), can be a pulsating sound caused by a blood vessel, bone disorders, a tumour, high blood pressure, muscle tension in the middle ear or neck, or a TMJ disorder. Sometimes there is a clicking sound due to muscle tension in the middle ear (tensor tympani, stapedius, tensor veli palatine muscles), Eustachian tube and/or a TMJ disorder. Subjective tinnitus is a sound that is experienced by only the person itself.

Diagnosis

Having a sound in the ear for more than six months can be considered as chronic.[100] Tinnitus is difficult to diagnose objectively because in most cases it is subjective tinnitus. There are CDs that contain selected tinnitus sounds and their strength from which the patient can select the sound and strength most close to what he or she perceives (to express to the outside world which sound he or

---

99 Han, B.I., Ho Won Lee, H.W., Kim, T.Y., Lim, J.S. and Shi, K.S., 'Tinnitus: characteristics, causes, mechanisms, and treatments', *Journal of Clinical Neurology* (2009) 5, 1, 11–19, www.ncbi.nlm.nih.gov/pmc/articles/PMC2686891 (accessed 10 August 2017).

100 Davis, A. and Refaie, A.E., 'Epidemiology of Tinnitus', in R.S. Tyler (ed.) *Tinnitus Handbook*, Singular Publishing Group, San Diego, CA, 2000.

she hears). The sound can be so loud and feel so very present that it drives people crazy, and very intense therapy might be needed to let the patient cope with the sound in general life because it can disturb a lot of pleasure and reduce the feeling of relaxation. It deranges the silence in the night, which is needed for a good and deep sleep; it can reduce focus on work or when socializing with friends because the sound may distract the attention. Sharp or high sounds – like the sound of a vacuum cleaner or a bathroom extractor fan – can be difficult to cope with because the ear can be (or become) very sensitive to sounds (*hyperacusis*).

Causes

- Barotrauma
- Ear inflammations
- Earwax
- Loss of hearing due to ageing
- Bridge angle tumour
- Infection of wisdom tooth
- Damage to hair cells of the inner ear due to exposure to loud noise
- Damage to middle or inner ear due to ear syringing
- Eustachian tube dysfunction
- Tension/spasm in the middle ear muscles
- Scalp and neck disorders (e.g. whiplash), trauma of the first rib
- TMJ disorders
- Problems in blood vessels
- Stress
- Hypertension
- Medication.

Tinnitus due to an underpressure or overpressure injury can occur when the round or oval window ruptures with a leak of perilymph as a result. Injuries of the windows can happen while descending (*implosion injury*) due to clearing too forcefully or while ascending in case the Eustachian tube is blocked (*explosion injury*). The tinnitus is experienced at the moment the injury happens or soon after the dive. Usually this tinnitus is combined with hearing loss or fullness of the affected ear and/or vertigo.

Due to my clinical experience I am convinced that many unexplained ear sounds have a mechanical cause and are the result of bruxism (clenching or teeth grinding) and/or related with high cervical-occipital problems (arthrogenic, muscular, blood circulation in the upper neck (i.e. C1–C3)). The combination of tinnitus and TMJ and high cervical-cranial problems frequently occurs in my practice and when treating the joint–muscle issues there usually is a reduction or total elimination of the tinnitus. It is not always easy to influence as, for example, TMJ disorders due to bruxism are difficult to break through as it is a habit related to controlling mechanisms and most of the time it is difficult for the patient to get rid of the controlling habit. But when the tinnitus is a symptom of TMJ and neck dysfunction you can be happy as a practitioner to have a gateway for the treatment, which is not the case when tinnitus is the result of damaged hair cells in the cochlea.

Dentists and orofacial physical therapists see temporomandibular disorders regularly combined with tinnitus. The auriculotemporal nerve or motor fibres of the mandibular nerve may be triggered, which may lead to tinnitus (see Section 2.2). The position of C1, for example, influences the position of the mandible: when C1 is positioned in extension it will shift the mandible forward; C1 standing in flexion shifts the mandible backwards. Extension or flexion of C1 will create tension in the jaw muscles.

If there are days or moments when the sound is not there, bruxism might be the cause. Clenching and teeth grinding are usually not done in the same way/intensity every night (*nocturnal bruxism*) – sometimes only just before awakening but very intense – and bruxism can occur seperately when awake (*awake bruxism*).

You can find out if the patient is clenching by, for example, asking him or her to perform a simple check in the morning when waking. The person has to feel with the tongue if there is a horizontal ridge at the inner side of the cheek. If so, it is obvious this person is clenching. This line disappears or reduces during the day. There are also people who clearly feel tension in the jaw muscles suddenly release when they wake up.

Some divers bite too hard in the mouthpiece of the regulator while diving, which can lead to muscle tension in the TMJ based on the same clenching mechanism.

People who gnash usually damage their teeth, for example flattening the incisors. A dentist is usually needed to diagnose gnashing and the resulting damage but I have seen patients with teeth where it was obvious they grinded (e.g. totally worn down lower teeth or completely flat incisors).

Extended research by an ENT doctor, a physiotherapist or an osteopath is required. It's not always that easy to find the cause of tinnitus as many factors can play a role and one mechanical issue can disturb a movement chain. Even a problem in a foot (for example limited extension in the big toe and/or hallux valgus) or an

SI (sacroiliac) joint problem can bring tension up the spine and to the TMJ. Also phlegm due to a common cold can clog the ears and trigger tinnitus.

An extended medical history and physical check often are needed to create an – as clear as possible – picture of the patient's functioning. Ask about traumas such as whiplash or falls, or whether the patient wore a dental brace in the past, which can also influence the TMJ. Examine the way your patient talks. Some people hardly move the jaws away from each other without realizing. Take a mirror to show them how they talk.

Our society, with lots of stress and pressure, easily results in muscle tension in the TMJ and neck. When there is a superficial high sternal breathing due to stress, a good and deep respiration – starting from the belly – can contribute to less tension of the muscles and fascia in the neck and decrease muscle traction at the ear and occiput.

Treatment

Often there is no targeted treatment offered but the advice is given that one should live with the tinnitus because there is insufficient scientific explanation about the cause.

Possible treatments are: relaxation therapy; wearing an ear mask; ignoring the sound; sedative medication when people have stress and/or insomnia due to the sound (e.g. benzodiazepines such as oxazepam, diazepam; or tricyclic antidepressants like amitriptyline); or in the case of noise damage corticosteroids (e.g. prednisone) combined with earplugs to try to calm the cochlear hair cells, applied as soon as possible after the noise damage. Zinc or vitamin B12 may support when there are demonstrated deficits.

If the tinnitus is caused by the TMJ, it can be helpful to wear a splint during the night to diminish the pressure in the TMJ, to do exercises to mobilize the TMJ, and to perform massage techniques on the jaw muscles, which can be done by the patient him or herself before sleeping. These massage techniques should be instructed clearly by a physiotherapist/physician. Experimental surgery might be performed if there is no other solution but this is very rare and generally only done with people who suffer for more than two or three years with a continuous sound.

If the trigger of tinnitus is temporomandibular joint disorder (TMD), the treatment may be very positive and helpful and it's possible to get rid of the TMD and the tinnitus totally, but it takes time to stop bruxism completely. The cause of the controlling habit has to be clear to solve it.

Chinese Medicine
Definition and Aetiology

Tinnitus or ringing in the ears (*Er Ming*) is a 'manifestation of functional impairment of hearing'.[101] It can lead to hearing loss (*Er Bei*) and deafness (*Er Long*).

In Chinese medicine tinnitus is traditionally divided into a deficiency (*Xu*) and an excess type (*Shi*). The deficiency type refers to the Kidney and the excess type is related to Liver and Gall Bladder-Fire or Phlegm-Heat. Due to my clinical experience I have added a Stagnation-type related to mechanical disorders (including injury) manifesting in stagnation of Qi and Xue. Examples of mechanical causes are a whiplash, TMJ disorders, middle ear and Eustachian tube dysfunction. In addition to excluding mechanical (TMJ and/or cervical spine) disorders, a very important indicator when diagnosing tinnitus is the pulse diagnosis to distinguish between the deficiency, excess and stagnation patterns as the sound can vary and therefore be difficult diagnostically.

Pattern Differentiation
1 Kidney Deficiency
- Clinical Signs and Symptoms

The Kidney sound is often intermittent and *low*; the sound can be like water flowing ('like holding a shell over the ear'[102]), a low buzz or low ringing, 'sometimes high pitched'[103] (when Kidney-Yin deficiency is combined with Liver-Yang rising[104]). The sound is often worse in the night. There is usually no acute occurrence of this tinnitus but a *gradual onset* as a result of the gradual emergence of the energy shortage. The sound might get less when the person puts pressure on the ear with a hand, which is not the case when there is an excess-type tinnitus (see Box 1.12.1). The Kidney opens into the ears and nourishes them.

When someone has a deficiency tinnitus, there may be typical Kidney weakness signs and symptoms like lower back or knee complaints. Overwork, excessive sexual activity, emotional strain (fear) and ageing weaken the Kidney. Besides the ear sound (more Yin deficient) there can be hearing loss too (more Yang deficient). Tinnitus due to deficiency might be worse when the person feels tired.

---

101 Geng, J.Y. and Su, Z.H., *Acupuncture and Moxibustion (Practical Traditional Chinese Medicine and Pharmacology)*, first edition, New World Press, Beijing, 1991.
102 Maclean, W. and Lyttleton, J., *Clinical Handbook of Internal Medicine*, Volume 1, fifth printing, University of Western Sydney, Sydney, 2008 (p.523).
103 Maclean, W. and Lyttleton, J., *Clinical Handbook of Internal Medicine*, Volume 1, fifth printing, University of Western Sydney, Sydney, 2008 (p.523).
104 Maciocia, G., *The Practice of Chinese Medicine: The Treatment of Diseases with Acupuncture and Chinese Herbs*, Churchill Livingstone, Edinburgh, 1994.

When there is Kidney-Yin deficiency there will be signs and symptoms of Five-palm Heat, night sweating and insomnia. In Kidney-Yang deficiency there will be cold signs and symptoms like feelings of coldness in the lower back and/or knees. In Kidney-Jing deficiency the signs and symptoms might be less distinctive.

Note: A low buzz can also be caused by pressure on a blood vessel, putting a strain on the blood circulation.

Pulse:

- Kidney-Yin deficiency: Thready (*Xi*) and Rapid (*Shuo*).
- Kidney-Yang deficiency: Deep (*Chen*), Thready (*Xi*) and Slow (*Chi*).
- Kidney-Jing deficiency: Deep (*Chen*), Thready (*Xi*) and Weak (*Ruo*).

Tongue:

- Kidney-Yin deficiency: Red and dry with a little or no coating.
- Kidney-Yang deficiency: Pale, swollen and wet.
- Kidney-Jing deficiency: Variable to more Yin or Yang deficiency.

● Treatment Principle

– Nourish and tonify Kidney-Yin, Kidney-Yang and/or Kidney-Jing.

– Open the ears.

● Acupuncture Points (select from)
KI-3 Taixi, **KI-6** Zhaohai, **CV-4** Guanyuan, **CV-6** Qihai, **GV-4** Mingmen, **BL-23** Shenshu, **KI-1** Yongquan, **TB-21** Ermen, **SI-19** Tinggong, **GB-2** Tinghui, **TB-17** Yifeng, YNSA Ear Point, Vertigo and Auditory Zone, Wrist Point 4, Ear Points: Inner Ear.C, Inner Ear.E.

● Explanation

- **KI-3**, **KI-6**, **CV-4**, **CV-6**, **GV-4**, **BL-23** and **KI-1** nourish and tonify the Kidney (for their different actions see Table 1.7.5).

    – Use moxa in the case of Kidney-Yang and Kidney-Jing deficiency.

- **TB-21**, **SI-19**, **GB-2** and **TB-17** benefit the ears and improve hearing acuity.

- YNSA Ear Point, Vertigo and Auditory Zone and Wrist Point 4 benefit the ears.

- Ear Points: Inner Ear.C and Inner Ear.E support the treatment. Use semi-permanent auricular needles.

> **BOX 1.12.1 DRUM OF THE HEAVEN**
>
> A massage exercise called *Drum of the Heaven* or *Open the Heaven´s Window* might help with reducing tinnitus caused by deficiency of the Kidney. Put the palms of the hands on the ears, apply pressure for two seconds and let go suddenly so you hear a *plopping* sound. Repeat over four minutes. This specific massage technique nourishes the ears and is performed at the China Beijing International Acupuncture Training Centre, China, where I learnt it in 2004.

- Food

Advice to affect Kidney-Yin tinnitus: no alcohol, coffee, tobacco or warming, pungent spices, because they give too much Heat. Soups, beans, seaweed, sea salt and blueberries support the Kidney.

2 Liver and Gall Bladder-Fire

- Clinical Signs and Symptoms

The sound related to Liver and Gall Bladder-Fire due to Liver-Qi stagnation is *high*, like 'the sounds of the drum or wind blowing'[105], a 'high pitched buzzing'[106] or a high-pitched beep. The ear can feel obstructed, distended or with a pressure inside.

The excess tinnitus usually has a *sudden* onset and is usually *continuous*.

Emotions that might be involved are anger, frustration, irritation, resentment, hate and stress. These disturbed emotions can cause Liver-Qi stagnation, which in the long term can evolve into Liver-Fire. There can be restlessness, insomnia, headache and constipation. The sound can be aggravated by an increase of emotions and stress. The face might be red.

Pulse: Wiry (*Xian*), Full (*Shi*) and Rapid (*Shuo*).

Tongue: Red or with red sides and a yellow coating.

- Treatment Principle

    — Clear Liver and Gall Bladder-Fire.

    — Calm the Shen.

    — Open the ears.

---

105 Geng, J.Y. and Su, Z.H., *Practical Traditional Chinese Medicine and Pharmacology, Acupuncture and Moxibustion*, first edition, New World Press, Beijing, 1991 (p.162).

106 Maclean, W. and Lyttleton, J., *Clinical Handbook of Internal Medicine*, Volume 1, fifth printing, University of Western Sydney, Sydney, 2008 (p.515).

EAR, NOSE AND THROAT DISORDERS

- **Acupuncture Points (select from)**
  LIV-2 Xingjian, **GB-43** Xiaxi, **GB-39** Xuanzong, **GB-20** Fengchi, **TB-5** Waiguan, **TB-3** Zhongzhu, **KI-1** Yongquan, **LIV-3** Taichong, **GB-42** Diwuhui, **LI-4** Hegu, **PC-6** Neiguan, **TB-21** Ermen, **SI-19** Tinggong, **GB-2** Tinghui, **TB-17** Yifeng, YNSA Ear Point, Vertigo and Auditory Zone, Wrist Point 4, Ear Points: Shenmen, Inner Ear.C, Inner Ear.E.

- **Explanation**

  - **LIV-2**, **GB-43** and **GB-39** clear Liver and Gall Bladder-Fire.
  - **GB-20**, **TB-5**, **TB-3** and **KI-1** subdue Liver-Yang and benefit the ears. In addition to affecting tinnitus **GB-20** and **TB-3** treat blocked ears.
  - **LI-4**–**LIV-3** combination or **PC-6** if there is long-term Liver-Qi stagnation.
  - **GB-42** spreads Liver-Qi and clears Gall Bladder-Heat (improves hearing and tinnitus).
  - **TB-21**, **SI-19**, **GB-2** and **TB-17** clear Heat, circulate Qi in the ear channels and benefit the ears.
  - YNSA Ear Point, Vertigo and Auditory Zone and Wrist Point 4 benefit the ears.
  - Ear Points: Shenmen calms the Shen; Inner Ear.C and Inner Ear.E benefit the ears.

- **Clinical Notes**

  - If someone cannot ground him or herself (*excess from the head*) and has tinnitus you can add **KI-1**, which subdues Liver-Yang and tonifies Kidney-Yin. When I needle this point, which can be very sensitive for the person, I push strongly with the thumb of my not-needling hand next to **KI-1** so that the needle is felt as little as possible (based on *two-points differentiation*).
  - As tinnitus can be hard to influence it might be necessary to use a combination of points, for example **GB-2**, **TB-17**, the YNSA Ear Point and **TB-3** in one treatment. Just adding a single point that benefits the ear is usually not enough.
  - The YNSA Ear Point is especially helpful in tinnitus. You can send the patient home with the needle still applied. Leave the needle in for about three hours. In most cases it supports reducing the intensity of the sound.

- The *Drum of Heaven* massage exercise does *not* diminish the strength of the sound in case of an excess tinnitus (see Box 1.12.1).

● Food

It is better to have no deep-fried food, coffee or alcohol because they may increase Liver-Fire. Water with lemon and mint tea clear the Heat of the Liver (some honey in the tea supports the Yin of the body).

3 Phlegm-Heat

● Clinical Signs and Symptoms

When there is Phlegm-Heat the sound is like cicadas[107, 108] or 'crickets'[109]. The sound of cicadas is higher than that of crickets. Excessive greasy and/or fried foods, irregular food intake, chronic worrying/excessive thinking or the intake of antibiotics cause Phlegm, which prevents the rising of clear Qi to the ears (*blocked orificia*). Often there is Spleen-Qi deficiency with Dampness underlying the Phlegm-Heat. Besides tinnitus there can be dizziness too. Phlegm can be accumulated in the Eustachian tube and middle ear with overstimulation of the inner ear.

Pulse: Slippery (*Hua*) and Rapid (*Shuo*).

Tongue: Red with a greasy yellow coating.

● Treatment Principle

- Transform Phlegm.
- Clear Heat.
- Open the ears.

● Acupuncture Points (select from)

ST-40 Fenglong, **ST-44** Neiting, **LI-11** Quchi, **SP-9** Yinlingquan, **CV-12** Zhongwan, **TB-3** Zhongzhu, **SP-6** Sanyinjiao, **ST-36** Zusanli, **TB-21** Ermen, **SI-19** Tinggong, **GB-2** Tinghui, **TB-17** Yifeng, **GB-20** Fengchi, YNSA Ear Point, Vertigo and Auditory Zone, Wrist Point 4, Ear Points: Inner Ear.C, Inner Ear.E.

---

107 Maclean, W. and Lyttleton, J., *Clinical Handbook of Internal Medicine*, Volume 1, fifth printing, University of Western Sydney, Sydney, 2008.

108 Maciocia G., *The Practice of Chinese Medicine, The Treatment of Diseases with Acupuncture and Chinese Herbs*, Churchill Livingstone, Edinburgh, 1994 (p.308).

109 Maciocia, G., *The Practice of Chinese Medicine: The Treatment of Diseases with Acupuncture and Chinese Herbs*, Churchill Livingstone, Edinburgh, 1994.

Explanation

- **ST-40** transforms Phlegm.

- **LI-11** and **ST-44** clear Heat.

- **SP-9** and **CV-12** transform Dampness (its resultant is Phlegm). **CV-12** affects Phlegm as well.

- **TB-3** is useful in the case of obstruction due to Phlegm-Heat. It is a strong working distal point for tinnitus. Instruct your patient to massage this point.

- **SP-6** and **ST-36** tonify the Spleen to prevent the formation of Phlegm.

- **TB-21**, **SI-19**, **GB-2** and **TB-17** clear Heat and Phlegm from the ear and benefit the ears.

- **GB-20** is very helpful for blocked ears.

- YNSA Ear Point, Vertigo and Auditory Zone and Wrist Point 4 benefit the ears.

- Ear Points: Inner Ear.C and Inner Ear.E support the treatment. Use semi-permanent auricular needles.

Clinical Notes

- **TB-21**[110] and **GB-2**[111] are particularly useful in the case of a *cricket sound*.

- According to Maciocia (2005), **ST-44** has as indications *aversion to the sound of people speaking* and *longing for silence*.[112]

Food

No cow's milk, sugar, coffee, alcohol, deep-fried or greasy foods. Grapefruit and pear have cooling properties and transform Phlegm.

4 Mechanical Causes of Tinnitus: Qi and Xue Stagnation
A. Cervical Spine Disorders

Cervical spine disorders can lead to tinnitus. Levine, quoted by Ramirez Aristeguieta, argues that 'Cervical muscular fatigue may produce tension on the vertebral artery which feeds the basilar artery and inner ear inflow, with

---

110 Ellis, A., Wiseman, N. and Boss, K., *Fundamentals of Chinese Medicine*, revised edition, Paradigm Publications, Brookline, MA, 2004.
111 Boermeester, W., *Tekstboek Acupunctuur, deel I, Punten*, Chinese Medicine Data, Kapellen, 1989.
112 Maciocia, G., *De Grondslagen van de Chinese Geneeskunde, Een Complete Basishandleiding voor Acupuncturisten en Fytotherapeuten, Tweede Uitgave*, Churchill Livingstone, New York, 2005.

exacerbated otic consequences'.[113] In this case tinnitus might be pulsating or sibilant and not continuous/daily depending of the tension in the cervical muscles and the mobility of the high cervical vertebrae.

The vertebral artery is located in the foramina transversia of the cervical spine. This artery enters the spine around C6. The vertebral artery provides blood to the basilar artery, which is located in the scalp. The basilar artery branches, among other locations, into the anterior inferior cerebellar artery, which divides again, among other locations, into the labyrinthine artery. The labyrinthine artery splits into the anterior vestibular artery which nourishes the vestibular organ and the common cochlear artery which supplies blood to the cochlea.

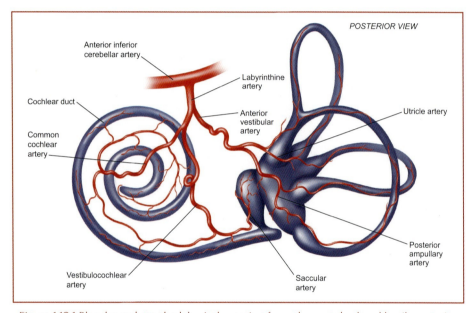

Figure 1.12.1 Blood supply to the labyrinth coming from the vertebral and basilar arteries

The sternocleidomastoid muscle is attached close to the high cervical spine (mastoid process of the temporal bone and the superior nuchal line of the occiput), which can pull at the ear region when there is muscle tension or muscle fatigue. The levator scapulae and scalenus anterior and medius muscles, which have their origins at the cervical spine, can influence the ear as well. The scalenus muscles have their insertion at the first rib and dislocation of this rib due to a trauma can influence the cervical spine by disturbed muscle function and muscle tension. Muscle tension and traction in the cervical region adversely affect the flow of Qi and Xue to the scalp, possibly resulting in tinnitus.

---

113 Ramirez Aristeguieta, L.M., Tinnitus and a Linked Stomatognathic System, in Fayez Bahmad (ed.) *Up to Date on Tinnitus*, InTech, Bogota, 2011 (p.49).

EAR, NOSE AND THROAT DISORDERS

- ● Clinical Signs and Symptoms
    - Stiffness of the neck, decreased range of motion (ROM)
    - Disposition of vertebrae (e.g. after a trauma) and reduced mobility in the facet joints
    - Muscle tension
    - Fixed pain (i.e. pain in a fixed location) and/or radiation of pain to and tingling sensations in the arms
    - There may be Ashi Points (including Trigger Points)
    - Possibly headache, vision problems, dizziness
    - Tinnitus (usually pulsating, sibilant, whizzing)
    - Emotional disbalance may be present (due to nerve stimulation).

    Pulse: Wiry (*Xian*) or Choppy (*Se*).

    Tongue: No signs (in the initial stage) or purple (or with purple stasis spots).

- ● Treatment Principle
    - Promote the circulation of Qi and Xue.
    - Benefit the muscles and facet joints.
    - Open the ears.

- ● Acupuncture Points (select from)
    SI-3 Houxi, **BL-62** Shenmai, **BL-10** Tianzhu, **GB-20** Fengchi, **GB-21** Jiangjing, **LI-4** Hegu, **LIV-3** Taichong, **SP-10** Xuehai, YNSA Basic A and Ear Points, Huatuo Jiaji Points, Ashi Points, **TB-21** Ermen, **SI-19** Tinggong, **GB-2** Tinghui, **TB-17** Yifeng, Vertigo and Auditory Zone, Wrist Point 4, Ear Points: Inner Ear.C, Inner Ear.E, Cervical Spine.

- ● Explanation
    - The combination **SI-3**–**BL-62** (Opening Points extraordinary vessel Du Mai) opens the Qi of the spine (decreases pain and stiffness).
    - **BL-10**, **GB-20** and **GB-21** benefit the neck. **BL-10** and **GB-20** especially influence occipital muscle tension. **GB-21** relaxes the trapezius muscle.
    - **LI-4**–**LIV-3** combination promotes the circulation of Qi and Xue.

- **SP-10** moves Xue.

- YNSA Basic A Point benefits the cervical spine (see Figure 1.7.3 and 'YNSA Basic Points' in Section 6.2).

- Huatuo Jiaji Points from the most fixed vertebral segments improve mobility and reduce muscle tension of the facet joints.

- Ashi Points (including Trigger Points) relieve pain and muscle tension.

- **TB-21**, **SI-19**, **GB-2** and **TB-17** benefit the ears, circulate Qi and Xue in the ear channels.

- YNSA Ear Point, Vertigo and Auditory Zone and Wrist Point 4 benefit the ears.

- Ear Points: Inner Ear.C, Inner Ear.E and Cervical Spine support the treatment.

- Ear candles support the circulation of Qi and Xue in the ear. Apply very carefully!

● Clinical Notes

- Huatuo Jiaji Points, also called *facet joint points*, are located 0.5 CUN lateral to the lower border of the spinous process of each vertebra of the spinal column. Needling the Huato Jiaji Points is a very effective way to treat facet joint blockages.

- Needling in the area around **GB-21** may improve the blood circulation through the vertebral and transverse cervical artery and can be useful in the case of insufficient cerebral blood circulation.[114]

- When you perform a (or a number of) mobilization technique(s) of the cervical spine/occiput zone and/or a short massage before needling you can achieve quicker recovery.

- Ear candles – made from very thin wax layers – can warm the external acoustic meatus. A light suction and the movement of the flame create a vibration of air in the ear candle and it will generate a massage-like effect on the tympanic membrane. This results in a very pleasant feeling of warmth and a balance in pressure in the ears.

---

114 Robinson, N.G., *Interactive Medical Acupuncture Anatomy*, Teton NewMedia, Jackson, WY, 2016.

B. TMJ Disorders (Liver-Qi Stagnation)

I have patients in my practice (diving and non-diving patients) who have tinnitus, but for whom the sound is not there every day. This implies that there is plausibly no damage in the inner ear and this kind of intermittent tinnitus is often due to bruxism (and cervical spine disorders as discussed already). Clenching and gnashing are usually not done with the same intensity every night. Depending on the existing muscle tone in the TMJ there might be an accompanying tinnitus. That means that nights with less or no clenching can result in having no tinnitus when awakening. There are also people who clench or move the mandible forwards in the day while focusing very intensely on their work or other occupation. Bruxism can cause TMJ dysfunction resulting in extreme tension in the jaw muscles, headache and stiffness of the neck. It is a habit that is usually not that easy to unlearn.

Several nerves, ligaments and muscles in the area around the TMJ have connections with the ear and Eustachian tube and might trigger tinnitus (see Section 2.2). In this section I will discuss tinnitus combined with TMJ disorders due to Liver-Qi stagnation.

● Clinical Signs and Symptoms

- Stiffness in the TMJ, decreased range of motion (difficulties opening the mouth), shift, snapping/clicking in the TMJ
- Tension in jaw muscles, involuntary rhythmic contractions of jaw-closing muscles (*chattering teeth*)
- Pain in the TMJ, which is aggravated by talking and/or chewing (*stomatognatic pain*); the pain might be described as *ear pain*
- Otic fullness, tinnitus
- Headache
- Stiffness of the neck
- Sighing
- Pellet-shaped stools.

Pulse: Wiry (*Xian*).

Tongue: No signs or dark (darkish sides or whole tongue).

● Treatment Principle

- Spread Liver-Qi.
- Benefit the TMJ.
- Open the ears.

DIVING MEDICAL ACUPUNCTURE

- **Acupuncture Points (select from)**
LI-4 Hegu, LIV-3 Taichong, PC-6 Neiguan, ST-6 Jiache, ST-7 Xiaguan, GB-2 Tinghui, SI-19 Tinggong, SI-17 Tianrong, ST-44 Neiting, Ashi Points, M-HN-9 Taiyang, TB-21 Ermen, TB-17 Yifeng, GB-20 Fengchi, GB-21 Jianjing, YNSA TMJ and Ear Points, Wrist Point 4, Vertigo and Auditory Zone, Ear Points: Inner Ear.C, Inner Ear.E, Shenmen and TMJ.

- **Explanation**
  - **LI-4–LIV-3** combination and **PC-6** spread Liver-Qi.
  - **ST-6**, **ST-7**, **GB-2**, **SI-19** and **SI-17** benefit the TMJ (pain, muscle tension, dislocation). **ST-6** improves the range of motion in the TMJ and alleviates tension or spasm of the masseter muscle. **ST-7**, **GB-2**, **SI-19** and **SI-17** also benefit the ears (tinnitus).
  - **ST-44** is an effective distal point to treat the TMJ. Especially good to use when the TMJ itself is too sensitive to needle.
  - Ashi Points (including Trigger Points) relieve pain and muscle tension.
  - Taiyang relaxes the temporalis muscle (temporal headache).
  - **TB-21** and **TB-17** circulate Qi in the ear channels and benefit the ears.
  - **GB-20** in the case of occipital headache or neck stiffness.
  - **GB-21** can be used if there is a Trigger Point found at this point.
  - YNSA TMJ and Ear Points and Wrist Point 4 benefit the TMJ and/or ear.
  - Vertigo and Auditory Zone benefits the ear in the case of tinnitus.
  - Ear Points: Inner Ear.C, Inner Ear.E, Shenmen and TMJ support the treatment.
  - Ear candles improve the circulation of Qi and Xue in the ear and TMJ region. Apply very carefully!

- **Clinical Notes**
  - A Trigger Point at **GB-21** forwards pain along the Gall Bladder channel (which closely passes the ear and TMJ by **GB-2**) to **TB-23** Sizhukong, **GB-1** Tongziliao and possibly some pain at **SI-17**. This Trigger Point can heighten myofascial dysfunction in the surrounding muscles and may result in headache, TMJ pain and stiffness in the neck.[115]

----

115 Robinson, N.G., *Interactive Medical Acupuncture Anatomy*, Teton NewMedia, Jackson, WY, 2016.

- When you perform a short massage of the jaw muscles before needling you can achieve quicker recovery. Massage before needling can also help the person relax physically and mentally. It especially can support when someone has bruxism due to mental stress caused by a need to feel in control. The massage shifts the focus to the body.

Food
Earl Grey tea and Omega 3 move Liver-Qi.

C. Barotrauma
Divers can get tinnitus due to an overpressure or underpressure injury. Damage can occur in the round or oval window with leakage of perilymph. The diver can have sudden deafness, vertigo and tinnitus when this trauma happens. Tinnitus due to the damaged structures might be irreversible. Surgery and/or rest are needed. Surgery should be done a week after a ruptured round or oval window. Acupuncture is not advised in the case of an acute ruptured window. When tinnitus does not diminish after the surgery you can treat the diver.

CASE STUDY 1.12.1 TINNITUS AFTER PERFORATION OF THE TYMPANIC MEMBRANE

Diver (31 years, female) with a perforated tympanic membrane (left ear) due to an underpressure injury.

Medical History
There was pain in the left ear for a short moment when descending (at 5 m depth) in the South Atlantic Ocean. As she was seasick the diver was focused on getting below the ocean waves as quickly as possible. She bit at the regulator feeling stressed due to the seasickness. The diver ignored the pain, which did not increase while descending more. After the dive there was blood and mucus in the mask. She went to a doctor who gave prednisone, antihistamines and a nose spray. Flying back home was no problem except that the ear felt obstructed; there was no pain. Five days after the injury the diver suddenly noticed tinnitus in the affected ear. The sound (high) was so loud that it was heard above everything else. She visited a diving medicine doctor who diagnosed a small perforation in the tympanic membrane and gave her another nose spray (Nasonex) to open the Eustachian tube. Two months later the diver contacted me for acupuncture hoping I would be able to help to get rid of the tinnitus. I mentioned several factors that could influence it:

- The diver had recurring common colds, which influenced ear-clearing, and there was chronic mucus production (probably due to daily intake of cow's milk and excessive thinking).

- The diver had high tension in the masseter and temporalis muscles affecting the left TMJ, which showed pressure sensitivity and having a shift while opening the mouth. The TMJ disorder probably occurred due to a high degree of work-related stress combined with testing lots of regulators professionally.

Chinese Medicine Diagnosis
Deficiency of Spleen Qi, Lung-Qi and Phlegm/Dampness.

Treatment
During four treatments I tonified the Spleen-Qi (**SP-3** Taibai, **SP-4** Gongsun, **SP-6** Sanyinjiao) and Lung-Qi (**LU-7** Lieque and **LU-9** Taiyuan), opened the nose (**LI-20** Yingxiang, **(EX)** Biyan), transformed Phlegm/Damp (**ST-40** Fenglong, **SP-9** Yinlingquan), relieved tension in the TMJ (temporalis muscle with **M-HN-9** Taiyang, masseter muscle with **ST-6** Jiache), opened the ear (**GB-2** Tinghui, **TB-17** Yifeng) and used the YNSA Ear Point for the tinnitus. Because of the busy lifestyle I needled **KI-3** Taixi and **CV-4** Guanyuan to support the basic energy. I advised to stop drinking cow's milk.

Result
The tinnitus changed into a sound only experienced at night in a totally silent surrounding, not disturbing the sleep, and also moments of having a silent ear. This positive improvement is an indication for some more treatments.

Table 1.12.1 Important acupuncture points to relieve (otic and somatic) tinnitus

Local points	Distal points	Special points/zones
TB-21 Ermen **SI-19** Tinggong **GB-2** Tinghui **TB-17** Yifeng **GB-20** Fengchi **ST-7** Xiaguan (TMJ)	**TB-3** Zhongzhu **GB-21** Jianjing (TMJ and neck) **LIV-2** Xingjian **GB-43** Xiaxi **GB-42** Diwuhui **ST-44** Neiting (TMJ) **KI-3** Taixi **KI-1** Yongquan	Auditory and Vertigo Zone YNSA Ear and TMJ Points Ear Points: Inner Ear.C, Inner Ear.E, TMJ, Shenmen, Wrist Point 4 In case of neck disorders: **SI-3** Houxi and **BL-62** Shenmai combination, **BL-10** Tianzhu, **GV-16** Fengfu, YNSA Basic A Point, Ashi Points (including Trigger Points)

EAR, NOSE AND THROAT DISORDERS

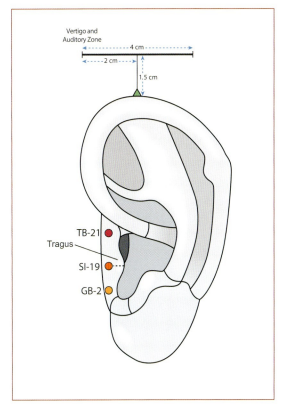

Figure 1.12.2 Local points to treat ear disorders

⬇ Advice for the Diver

- Always visit a Western physician first when you have tinnitus and try to find the cause of it. Jaw problems accompanying tinnitus often present as *pain in the ear*. If there are neck or jaw problems it's advisable to visit a manual therapist, physiotherapist or an osteopath as well.

- Prevent diving situations that may give you a lot of stress, such as drift dives or cave diving. Stress might influence the sound due to muscle tension.

- Don't drink coffee before a dive because it increases the adrenalin level and the feeling of stress (an increase in heartbeat, breathing and muscle tension), and it might aggravate the ear sound.

- Learn some relaxation techniques and exercises with a specialist/physiotherapist.

- Be sure the mouthpiece of your regulator fits well in your mouth. There are several sizes of mouthpiece available (smaller, longer and/or shorter) that will fit on most regulators. You also can have one specially made to fit the size of your mouth, available at any dive shop.

- When you clench while sleeping, a splint can be helpful to relax the TMJ and to protect the teeth. The splint can be made by a dentist or a jaw surgeon. X-rays of the TMJ are advised to exclude other pathology.

- Don't eat chewing gum, potato crisps or nuts to prevent one-point pressure on the teeth, or whole apples (it is better to cut the apples into small pieces) because the mouth has to be opened too wide. French bread and pizza are often too difficult to chew. When the jaw problem is solved you can carefully try some of these products but the advice is not to chew like a cow for hours on the grass…because that might trigger the sound again.

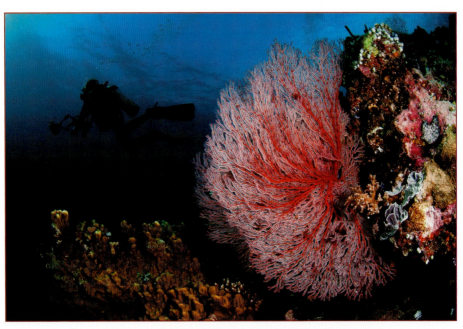

Figure 1.12.3 Janneke Vermeulen with her underwater camera in the Western Pacific Ocean, Palau, Micronesia, 2011
Photo: Dr Simon Mitchell from New Zealand (anaesthesiologist, specialist in diving and hyperbaric medicine)

CHAPTER 2

TEMPOROMANDIBULAR JOINT DISORDERS
颞下颌关节疾患

2.1 TEMPOROMANDIBULAR JOINT DISORDER AND THE REGULATOR
颞下颌关节疾患和调节器

Diving implies that you are under water with a regulator in your mouth to be able to breathe air. In the past the mouthpiece of the regulator was a one-size item and often quite large. This could mean that the mouthpiece did not fit well in every mouth. Nowadays every brand provides smaller mouthpieces too as it's very important to have a mouthpiece of the right size. There are even brands that supply mouthpieces that can be made especially for one specific person. This is done by immersing the standard mouth part in boiling water for a couple of seconds, then putting it in your mouth and biting for a while so the mouth part will adapt to the shape of your teeth/mouth. The company Mares, for example, supplies the *Mares JAX* and *Mares JAX-S* (a small version), which were developed in the dental industry.

When the mouthpiece of the regulator is too large the diver will clench to prevent the regulator slipping out of the mouth. This results in tension of the jaw muscles. A mouthpiece that is too small can be uncomfortable because it can shift in the mouth. In that case you have to clamp to keep it in the right place.

When there is strong current you may bite harder on your regulator because otherwise the current will push the regulator out of your mouth. In these circumstances some clamping is needed not to lose the regulator.

In general scuba divers who are dealing with anxiety bite more on their regulator than divers who are relaxed and are feeling comfortable in the underwater surroundings. Some divers really destroy the mouthpiece of their regulator because they bite extremely hard. People who clamp can have a headache or TMJ pain after the dive because the temporomandibular joint is overloaded. Tension in the masseter and/or temporalis muscles might be clearly visible (swelling).

2.2 TEMPOROMANDIBULAR JOINT DISORDER AND TINNITUS
颞下颌关节疾患和耳鸣

Western Medicine

Definition and Aetiology

Temporomandibular joint disorder (TMD or TMJD) is an arthrogenic (relating to ligaments, capsule, synovium, discus, cartilage, bone) and/or muscular disorder.

The temporomandibular joint itself comprises:

- a capsule and articular surfaces
- an articular disc and retrodiscal tissue
- muscles
- ligaments.

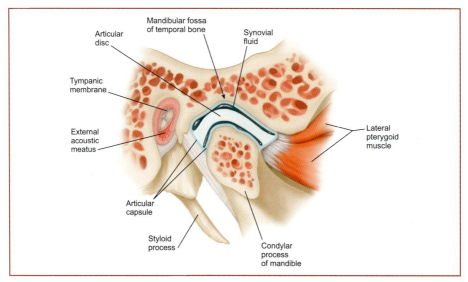

Figure 2.2.1 Side view of the temporomandibular joint. The external acoustic meatus and middle ear are positioned very closely to the TMJ. This is why people often say they have ear pain when it is TMJ pain

The muscles of the TMJ are:

- temporalis muscle
- masseter muscle
- medial and lateral pterygoid muscles
- digastric muscle.

TEMPOROMANDIBULAR JOINT DISORDERS

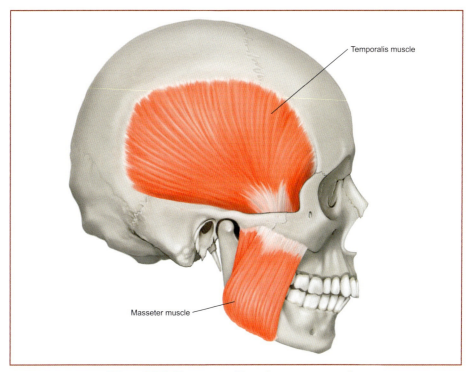

Figure 2.2.2 The temporalis and masseter muscles

The ligaments of the TMJ are:

- discomalleolar ligament (or discomallear ligament, Pinto's ligament)
- anterior mandibular ligament (or malleomandibular ligament)
- temporomandibular ligament (or lateral ligament)
- stylomandibular ligament
- sphenomandibular ligament.

The muscles make the movements and the ligaments provide passive stability to the TMJ. The discomalleolar and the anterior mandibular ligaments are also called the *otomandibular ligaments* because they connect the malleus in the middle ear with the TMJ (see Figure 2.2.3).

Nerves, Muscles and Ligaments Around the TMJ and Tinnitus

- The trigeminal ganglion is the sensory ganglion of the trigeminal nerve (V), which has his origin close to the temporomandibular joint. The trigeminal nerve divides into the ophthalmic (V1), maxillary (V2) and mandibular (V3) nerves.

- The mandibular nerve is a motor and sensory nerve, in contrast to the ophthalmic and maxillary nerves, which are only sensory. The mandibular branch divides into, among others, the auriculotemporal nerve (which regulates sensory innervation of the external ear (skin), the tympanic membrane and TMJ capsule) *and* into motor branches, which activate the tensor tympani and tensor veli palatine muscles.

- The trigeminal ganglion or parts of the trigeminal nerve, and specifically, the mandibular nerve, can be irritated in TMJ disorders.

In my clinical experience TMJ disorders are frequently the cause of *unexplained tinnitus* or, rather, *underdiagnosed tinnitus,* as tinnitus in combination with TMJ disorders diminishes or disappears by treating the TMJ.

Scientifically tinnitus raises lots of questions in respect of possible causes of this intricate *symptom*; there are no efficient medications and we have to work with some assumptions regarding the potential causes. However, the current neural, muscular, ligamentary and vascular theories suggesting a link between TMJ dysfunction and tinnitus look quite logical besides being complicated as well.

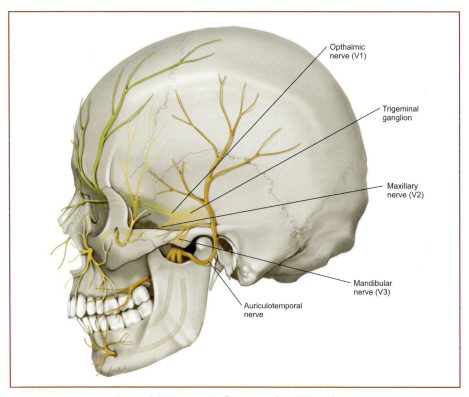

Figure 2.2.3 Nerves influencing the TMJ and ear

BOX 2.2.1 THEORIES ABOUT THE ONSET OF TINNITUS

- Costen (quoted by Kaan Beriat, Celebi Beriat and Uysal) explained in 1934 that disposition of the condyle of the mandible to the posterior can compress the auriculotemporal nerve and the chorda tympani nerve.[1]

- An abnormally stimulated auriculotemporal nerve might produce 'reflex vascular spasm in the labyrinthine system'.[2]

- Overstimulation of the trigeminal ganglion, which can happen in TMD, can affect the blood flow in the inner ear through the basilar and anterior inferior cerebellar arteries.[3]

- The trigeminal ganglion innervates the vascular supply of the dorsal and ventral cochlear nucleus and the superior olivary complex (cerebral parts of the auditory system).[4]

- Dysfunction of the tensor tympani and the tensor veli palatini muscles due to TMD might cause tinnitus by affecting the middle ear and Eustachian tube.[5,6]

- The discomalleolar and anterior mandibular ligaments are connected with the malleus in the middle ear and when stretched in the case of TMD, they can cause otic symptoms (tinnitus, vertigo, earache).[7]

- Von Piekartz (2007) explains that pulling forces from Pinto's ligament (discomalleolar ligament) at the malleus trigger the vestibulocochlear nerve ('depolarization') during movements of the mandible (protrusion and laterotrusion) and they 'can change the qualities of the frequency of the tinnitus'.[8]

---

1   Kaan Beriat, G., Celebi Beriat, N. and Uysal, S., 'Relationship between somatic tinnitus and temporomandibular joint dysfunction signs and symptoms', *Clinical Dentistry and Research* (2011) 35, 1, 26.
2   Ramirez, A.L.M., Sandoval, O.G.P. and Ballesteros, L.E., 'Theories on otic symptoms in TMD: Past and present', *International Journal of Morphology* (2005) 23, 2, 141–156 (p.146).
3   Ramirez Aristeguieta, L.M., 'Tinnitus and a Linked Stomatognathic System', in Fayez Bahmad (ed.) *Up to Date on Tinnitus*, InTech, Bogota, 2011.
4   Ramirez Aristeguieta, L.M., 'Tinnitus and a Linked Stomatognathic System', in Fayez Bahmad (ed.) *Up to Date on Tinnitus*, InTech, Bogota, 2011.
5   Ramirez, A.L.M., Sandoval, O.G.P. and Ballesteros, L.E., 'Theories on otic symptoms in TMD: Past and present', *International Journal of Morphology* (2005) 23, 2, 141–156.
6   Schames, J., Schames, M. and Boyd, J.P., 'Trigeminal pharyngioplasty: Treatment of the forgotten accessory muscles of mastication which are associated with orofacial pain and ear symptomology', *Journal of Pain Management* (2002) 12, 3, 102–112.
7   Ramirez, A.L.M., Sandoval, O.G.P. and Ballesteros, L.E., 'Theories on otic symptoms in TMD: Past and present', *International Journal of Morphology* (2005) 23, 2, 141–156.
8   Pieckartz, H.J.M. von, *Craniofacial Pain, Neuromusculoskeletal Assessment, Treatment and Management*, Elsevier, Edingurgh, 2007 (pp.473–474).

- One-sided tinnitus can be associated with TMJ disc displacement.[9]
- An interrupted blood flow between the TMJ and middle ear due to TMD may influence the auditory system.[10]

Somatic and Otic Tinnitus

Levine (1999) explained *craniocervical* tinnitus as 'a somatic auditory perception interference [a somatic pathway] in the dorsal (DCN) and ventral cochlear nucleus by trigeminal innervation'.[11] He named it *somatic tinnitus* as the cause of the tinnitus is located outside the ear (e.g. whiplash, TMJ disorder).

Levine suggests benzodiazepines like Valium (diazepam) and Clonex or Klonopin (clonazepam) to quieten the tinnitus as it is helpful in about 75 per cent of tinnitus patients by reducing muscle tension and anxiety/fear. Its effect is dose-related and works within a few minutes to hours. Side-effects are sedation and imbalance.[12] These side-effects are contraindications for diving so other solutions like acupuncture and physiotherapy are advisable. Levine's research makes clear that relaxation of the muscles in the TMJ and neck region can reduce the intensity of the tinnitus.

In addition to somatic tinnitus there is *otic tinnitus*. Otic tinnitus is 'inner ear originated tinnitus' caused by damage of the cochlear hair cells due to ageing or to an acoustic trauma (sound, music).[13] The vestibulocochlear nerve (VIII) triggers the dorsal cochlear nucleus located in the brainstem (an otic pathway).

As reported by Baguley (2000), 'Levine hypothesised that decreases in inhibitory MSN input to the DCN (specifically inhibition) might result in disinhibition of DCN activity leading to increased activity and the perception of tinnitus' (see Figure 2.2.4).[14]

---

9   Ren, Y.F. and Isberg, A., 'Tinnitus in patients with temporomandibular joint internal derangement', *Cranio* (1995) 13, 2, 75–80.
10 Ramirez Aristeguieta, L.M., Tinnitus and a Linked Stomatognathic System, in Fayez Bahmad (ed.) *Up to Date on Tinnitus*, InTech, Bogota, 2011, p.37.
11 Levine, R.A., 'Somatic (craniocervical) tinnitus and the dorsal cochlear nucleus hypothesis', *American Journal of Otolaryngology* 1999, 20:351–362.
12 Levine, R.A., *Clonazepam (Klonopin) for Tinnitus*, https://docs.google.com/viewer?a=v&pid=sites&srcid =ZGVmY XVsdGRvbWFpbnxkb2N0b3JsZXZpbmVzdGlubml0dXNzaXRlIf Gd4OjQ5OGU3M2M0 NDY1NjM0YTU (accessed 14 September 2017).
13 Levine, R.A., 'Somatic (craniocervical) tinnitus and the dorsal cochlear nucleus hypothesis', *American Journal of Otolaryngology* (1999) 20, 351–362.
14 Baguley, D.M., 'Mechanisms of tinnitus,' *British Medical Bulletin* (2002) 63, 195–212, p.206.

TEMPOROMANDIBULAR JOINT DISORDERS

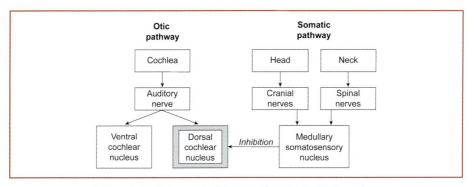

Figure 2.2.4 Schematic diagram of suggested interaction between the somatic and otic pathways (following Levine)
Source: Baguley (2000), reproduced with kind permission of Oxford University Press.[15]

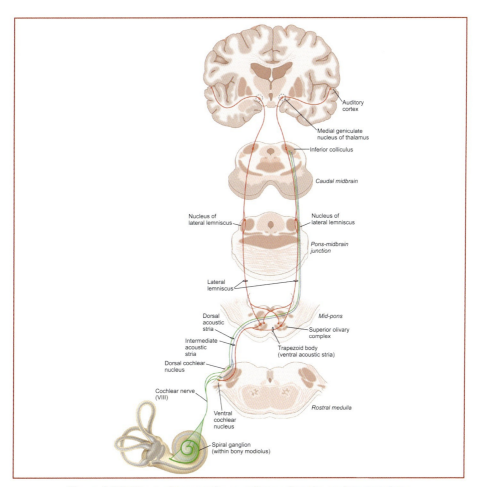

Figure 2.2.5 The auditory pathway: all neural paths and connections between the cochlea and the auditory cortex

• • • • • • • • • • • • • • • • • • •
15 Baguley, D.M., 'Mechanisms of tinnitus,' *British Medical Bulletin* (2002) 63, 195–212, p.206.

Tensor Tympani and Tensor Veli Palatini Muscles

The tensor tympani muscle (TTM) is an important muscle to reduce the intensity of sound from chewing, vocalization and external stimuli. The tensor veli palatine muscle (TVPM) opens the Eustachian tube while swallowing and yawning, and ventilates the middle ear. The TT and TVP muscles are innervated by branches of the mandibular nerve (V3). TMD can irritate the motor fibres of the mandibular nerve with activation of the innervated muscles as a result. According Ramirez, Sandoval and Ballesteros (2005) both muscles are attached to the handle of the malleus. Therefore they 'act synergistically together and temporary can increase intra-tympanic pulling force with otic symptoms like otalgia, tinnitus, vertigo and subjective hearing loss'.[16]

BOX 2.2.2 TEMPOROMANDIBULAR JOINT DISORDER

'TMD may produce constant (spastic) or episodic (clonic) contraction and tension of the TT and TVP muscles during a state of fatigue.' (Ramirez 2011)[17]

Divers and Non-Divers

Some divers bite too hard at the mouthpiece of the regulator, which results in increased tension in the TMJ with possibly stimulation of the mandibular nerve and the TT/TVP muscles and associated muscle tension, spasm or fatigue. Clenching at the mouthpiece often leads to equalizing problems. According to Bluestone (2005) an inefficiently working TVP muscle will not effectively open the Eustachian tube[18] and this could explain why clearing the ears while clenching does not succeed.

Non-divers with tinnitus who clench in the day due to focusing or stress, or clench/gnash during sleep, can irritate the mandibular nerve and the TT/TVP muscles in the same way. The treatment given here is suitable for them as well. Stress can quickly influence the tension in the TMJ. People who clench the jaw often suffer from migraines due to tension in the masseter or temporalis muscles.

---

16 Ramirez, A.L.M., Sandoval, O.G.P. and Ballesteros, L.E., 'Theories on otic symptoms in TMD: Past and present', *International Journal of Morphology* (2005) 23, 2, 141–156 (p. 145).

17 Ramirez Aristeguieta, L.M., 'Tinnitus and a Linked Stomatognathic System', in Fayez Bahmad (ed.) *Up to Date on Tinnitus*, InTech, Bogota, 2011 (p.22).

18 Bluestone, C.D., *Eustachian Tube: Structure, Function, Role in Otitis Media*, BD Decker Inc., Lewiston, NY, 2005.

TEMPOROMANDIBULAR JOINT DISORDERS

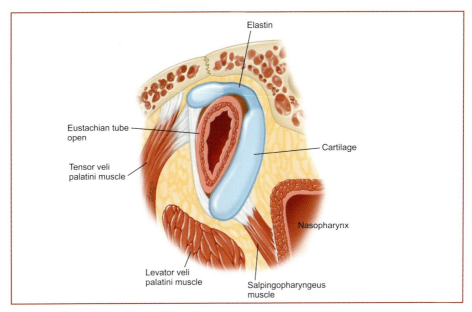

Figure 2.2.6a The tensor veli palatini muscle opens the Eustachian tube while swallowing or yawning and ventilates the middle ear

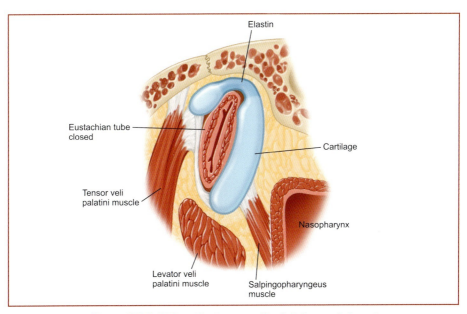

Figure 2.2.6b When the tensor veli palatini muscle is not contracted the Eustachian tube will be closed

2.3 MUSCLES AND LIGAMENTS OF THE TMJ AND MIDDLE EAR
和中耳的肌肉和肌腱

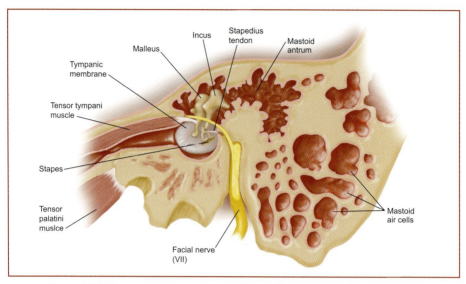

Figure 2.3.1 The tensor tympani, stapedius and tensor veli palatini muscles

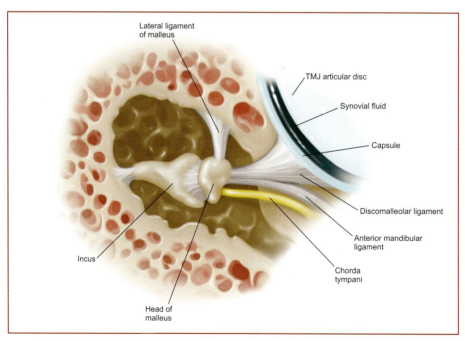

Figure 2.3.2 Discomalleolar and anterior mandibular ligaments. These ligaments connect the malleus with the articular disc of the TMJ and the mandible. For clarity only the relevant structures are shown in this view. The tympanic membrane is located to the right of the lateral ligament of the malleus behind the bony structure

The attachments, functions and innervations of the TMJ and middle ear muscles and the TMJ ligaments are described below to support the understanding of TMJ disorders and its possible and complex relation with tinnitus. This understanding means your acupuncture treatment can be more focused on the origin of the condition if there is a physical factor.

Masseter Muscle

Origin: Zygomatic arch and maxillary process of the zygomatic bone.

Insertion: Lateral surface of the ramus of the mandible.

Function: Elevation of the mandible (closes the mouth).

Innervation: Masseteric nerve from the mandibular division (V3) of the trigeminal nerve (V).

Temporalis Muscle

Origin: Bone of the temporal fossa and temporal fascia.

Insertion: Coronoid process of the mandible and anterior border of the ramus of the mandible, almost as far as the last molar tooth.

Function: Elevation and retraction of the mandible (closes the mouth).

Innervation: Deep temporal nerves from the mandibular division (V3) of the trigeminal nerve (V).

Medial Pterygoid Muscle

Origin: Tuberosity of the maxilla and pyramidal process of the palatine bone (superficial head) and pterygoid process and pyramidal process of the palatine bone (deep head).

Insertion: Medial surface of the ramus of the mandible near the angle.

Function: Elevation and laterotrusion of the mandible (closes the mouth).

Innervation: Medial pterygoid nerve from the mandibular division (V3) of the trigeminal nerve (V).

Lateral Pterygoid Muscle

Origin: Roof of the infratemporal fossa of the sphenoid bone (upper head) and lateral surface of the lateral plate of the pterygoid process (lower head).

Insertion: Capsule and disc of TMJ (upper head) and pterygoid fovea on the neck of the mandible (lower head).

Function: Protrusion and laterotrusion of the mandible, brings the discus forward (opens the mouth).

Innervation: Lateral pterygoid nerve of the mandibular division (V3) of the trigeminal nerve (V).

Digastric Muscle

Origin: Digastric fossa of the mandible (anterior belly), mastoid notch on the mastoid process of the temporal bone (posterior belly).

Insertion: Hyoid bone.

Function: Depression of the mandible, elevation of the hyoid (opens the mouth).

Innervation: Anterior belly by the mandibular division (V3) of the trigeminal nerve (V) and the posterior belly by the facial nerve (VII).

Tensor Tympani Muscle

Origin: Cartilaginous and bony margins of the Eustachian tube and the adjoining part of the greater wing of the sphenoid.

Insertion: Upper part of the handle of the malleus.

Function: Pulls the handle of the malleus medially (pushes the stapes into the oval window), tenses the tympanic membrane (reduces the intensity of sounds).

Innervation: Branch from the mandibular division (V3) of the trigeminal nerve (V).

Stapedius Muscle

Origin: Inside of pyramidal eminence.

Insertion: Neck of the stapes.

Function: Pulls the stapes posteriorly, prevents excessive oscillation (reduces the intensity of sounds).

Innervation: Branch of the facial nerve (VII).

Tensor Veli Palatini Muscle

Origin: Scaphoid fossa of the sphenoid bone, spine of sphenoid and fibrous part of the Eustachian tube.

Insertion: Palatine aponeurosis.

Function: Tenses the soft palate, opens the Eustachian tube during swallowing and yawning (important for clearing the ears).

Innervation: Via the nerve to the medial pterygoid muscle from the mandibular division (V3) of the trigeminal nerve (V).

Discomalleolar Ligament

Origin: Malleus.

Insertion: The retrodiscal tissue of the TMJ.

Function: Limits protrusion of the disc.

Anterior Mandibular Ligament

Origin: Malleus.

Insertion: Lingula of the mandible (via the sphenomandibular ligament).

Function: The function of this ligament is not clear. Excessive forces on the mandible and this ligament may lead to dislocation of the ossicles.[19]

Temporomandibular Ligament

This ligament is the thickened lateral part of the TMJ capsule and is divided into an outer oblique section and an inner horizontal section.

Origin: Zygomatic bone.

Insertion: Mandible condyl.

Function: Limits retraction of the condyle and disc (outer oblique section) and rotational movement (inner horizontal section).

---

19   Gola, R., Chossegros, C. and Cheynet, F., 'Oto-mandibular ligaments: Disco-mallear and malleo-mandibular ligaments', *Revue de stomatologie et de chirurgie maxillo-faciale* (1997) 98, 2, 66–71.

Stylomandibular Ligament

Origin: Styloid process.

Insertion: Angle of the mandible.

Function: Limits protrusion of the mandible.

Sphenomandibular Ligament

Origin: Spine of the sphenoid bone.

Insertion: Lingula of the mandible.

Function: Limits protrusion of the mandible.

CASE STUDY 2.3.1 MIGRAINE DUE TO TMJ DISORDER

I treated a patient (male, 25 years) who had unexplained migraines for eight years.

Medical History
The attacks occurred twice a week and he had to use Imigran by injection for every migraine attack. One of the causes of his TMJ disorder was the very poor condition of his teeth, which had to be extracted by his dentist. Besides the dental issue there was a lot of stress in general, which resulted in high muscle tension of the temporalis muscle.

Chinese Medicine Diagnosis
Liver-Qi stagnation.

Treatment
The treatment was focused on relaxation in general (**LI-4** Hegu, **LIV-3** Taichong, Ear Point: Shenmen, **M-HN-3** Yintang) and in the TMJ (**M-HN-9** Taiyang, **ST-7** Xiaguan, Ashi points, YNSA TMJ Point; Ear Point: TMJ Point); additionally, the YNSA Basic A Point was used to alleviate the migraine itself. Before needling I massaged the temporalis and masseter muscles.

Result
After eight acupuncture treatments he was totally free of the complaint.

2.4 TMJ DISORDERS
颞下颌关节疾患

Western Medicine

TMJ disorders can be differentiated into:[20]

- inflammatory disorders (capsulitis, synovitis, retrodiscitis)
- internal structural changes like dislocation of the disc due to hypermobility, or wearing a brace[21]
- muscular disorders (tension, spasm)
- hypermobility
- degenerative disorders (osteoarthritis).

Aetiology

- Bruxism (grinding teeth or clenching). People who grind during the night usually clench during the day. Clenching teeth is the same mechanically as biting on the mouthpiece of a regulator. Clenching often has an emotional cause, such as a need to control things in one's life or when focusing/concentrating on something very much. Divers may clench when they feel stressed or are worried that they will not be able to clear their the ears while descending. Bruxism can be triggered by having parasites in the liver and intestines as well as the release of toxins.

- Mouth breathing due to a blocked nose. When the mouth is opened, the tongue is positioned downwards, on the bottom of the mouth, which brings the TMJ out of position. This results in tension in the jaw muscles and possibly pain in the TMJ. When breathing through the nose the tongue is positioned on the top of the mouth against the upper arch. Nose breathing takes more effort than mouth breathing but means that the air is filtered, warmed and moistened and fluids in the nasal cavity and sinuses can be transported to the throat. Mouth breathing can result in accumulation of fluids in the nose and sinuses and contribute to infections and inflammation. Mouth breathing can be accompanied by a very dry mouth (especially when awakening), a foggy head in the morning, gum and teeth problems, bad breath, a recessed chin, headache,

---

20 Mark, B.M., 'Common disorders of the temporomandibular joint', *Acupuncture Today* (2014) 15, 3. B.M. Mark and C.S. Kessler, *All Pain Is Not the Same: A Unique Perspective on Headaches, TMJ Disorders and Facial Pain*, Jimsam Inc. Publishing, Lobelville, TN, 2011.

21 Own clinical experience.

dizziness, tinnitus, immune disfunction, cardiac arrhythmia, indigestion, sleep apnoea, insomnia and chronic fatigue.

- Hard chewing (nuts, pizza, baguette).
- Lots of chewing (chewing gum, potato crisps) with one point of contact.
- Pressing the lips together.
- Opening the mouth too wide (e.g. when eating an apple, having a regulator with a mouthpiece that is too large, dental treatment where the mouth is wide open and the neck extended for a long period).
- An external trauma (whiplash, external force against the mandible, e.g. when boxing).
- Spine disorders. When the scalp and C1 are standing in extension the mandible will shift forward; when the scalp and C1 are positioned in flexion the mandible is pushed backwards. An SI blockage also may cause tension in the whole spine and the TMJ.
- Even foot problems can influence the tension in the TMJ. When someone has pes planovalgus or a hallux valgus every step the person takes might cause an increase of muscle tension in the TMJ. If there are foot problems it might be wise to visit a podiatrist (besides that, it's recommended to perform excersis to support the posture of the foot). There are orthotics you can put in your diving shoes when you need to walk longer distances before you go into the water. It's necessary to make them the same length as your diving shoes because when they are shorter they will float to the front of your diving shoes when you get out of the water and then it's difficult walking back…

> ### BOX 2.4.1 RELATIONSHIP OF BLOCKED NOSE TO TMJ AND EAR DISORDERS
>
> Blocked nose ➔ Mouth breathing ➔ TMJ disorder ➔ Ear disorder
>
> Chronic mouth breathing due to a blocked nose is an ENT disorder that can cause a TMJ disorder, possibly resulting in tinnitus.

Treatment

Correct the position and the movements of the mandible; relax the jaw muscles (during opening the mouth it is visible and palpable when the mandible shifts). If there is bruxism it can be helpful to wear a *resin splint* in the night until the bruxism is cured. The splint will protect the teeth, gives feedback (makes you conscious of the bruxism) and offers optimal balanced contact. With the splint the TMJ can't be closed totally so there is less pressure in the joints. It is important that the splint is not too thick: it should be possible to close the mouth in a relaxed way. Some people clench so strongly that they even bite the splint into pieces. Consequently relaxation techniques (*habit reversal*) are very important in changing this difficult habit.

Chinese Medicine
Definition and Aetiology

In Chinese medicine temporomandibular disorder is seen as an 'oral disease'.[22] It is characterized by (1) pain, (2) tenderness, (3) swelling and (4) discomfort in one or both sides of the temporomandibular joint at rest and when opening or closing the mouth, and is worsened by yawning, chewing and/or talking.

When there is 'snapping or popping of the joint' we call this 'articular dyskinesia'.[23]

As a result of the temporomandibular disorder there may be other complaints such as neck pain, headache, facial pain and tinnitus. TMJ pain is often described as *ear pain* due to its close proximity to the ear. The jaw region is energetically associated with the Liver. Bruxism is called *Nie Chi*.

Dysfunction of the temporomandibular joint in Chinese medicine is traditionally divided into:[24]

- mandibular pain or He Tong
- cheek pain or Jia Tong
- lockjaw or Kou Jin Bu Kai.

Pattern Differentiation

1 Liver-Qi Stagnation

Liver-Qi flow problems due to stress, anxiety or anger can result in stiffness of the jaw muscles.

---

22 Yin, G. and Liu, Z., *Advanced Modern Chinese Acupuncture Therapy*, New World Press, Beijing, 2000 (p.518).
23 Yin, G. and Liu, Z., *Advanced Modern Chinese Acupuncture Therapy*, New World Press, Beijing, 2000 (p.518).
24 Yin, G. and Liu, Z., *Advanced Modern Chinese Acupuncture Therapy*, New World Press, Beijing, 2000.

- Clinical Signs and Symptoms

    - Stiffness in the TMJ, decreased range of motion (difficulties opening the mouth), shifting, snapping/clicking in the TMJ
    - Tension in the jaw muscles, involuntary rhythmic contractions of jaw-closing muscles (*chattering teeth*)
    - Pain in the TMJ, which is aggravated by talking and/or chewing (*stomatognatic pain*); pain might be described as ear pain
    - Otic fullness, possibly tinnitus
    - Pain or tingling in the face
    - Headache
    - Muscle tension in the high cervical/occipital region and/or stiffness of the neck
    - Sighing
    - Pellet-shaped stools.

    Pulse: Wiry (*Xian*).

    Tongue: No signs (in the initial stage) or dark (darkish sides or whole tongue).

- Treatment Principle

    - Spread Liver-Qi.
    - Benefit the TMJ.
    - Calm the Shen.

- Acupuncture Points (select from)

    LI-4 Hegu, **LIV-3** Taichong, **PC-6** Neiguan, **ST-6** Jiache, **ST-7** Xiaguan, **GB-2** Tinghui, **SI-19** Tinggong, **SI-17** Tianrong, **GB-20** Fengchi, **GB-21** Jianjing, **ST-44** Neiting, Ashi Points, **M-HN-9** Taiyang, YNSA TMJ and Ear Points, Ear Points: Shenmen and TMJ.

- Explanation

    - **LI-4–LIV-3** combination and **PC-6** spread Liver-Qi.
    - **ST-6**, **ST-7**, **GB-2**, **SI-19** and **SI-17** benefit the TMJ (pain, muscle tension, dislocation). **ST-6** improves the range of motion in the TMJ and alleviates tension or spasm of the masseter muscle. **ST-7**, **GB-2**, **SI-19** and **SI-17** also benefit the ears (tinnitus).

- **GB-20** in the case of occipital headache or stiffness of the neck.

- **GB-21** can be used if a Trigger Point is found at this point (see 'Clinical Notes' in Section 1.12.4.B).

- **ST-44** is an effective distal point to treat the TMJ. Especially good to use when the TMJ itself is too sensitive to needle.

- Ashi Points (including Trigger Points) relieve pain and muscle tension.

- Taiyang relaxes the temporalis muscle (temporal headache).

- YNSA TMJ Point benefits the TMJ. If there is tinnitus due to the tension in the TMJ region you can add the YNSA Ear Point.

- Ear Points: Shenmen calms the Shen and the TMJ Point benefits the TMJ in general.

● Clinical Notes

- When you perform a short massage of the jaw muscles before needling you can achieve quicker recovery. Due to the massage the person also can be physically and mentally relaxed before needling. This can support someone especially when he or she has bruxism due to mental stress. The massage shifts the focus to the body.

CASE STUDY 2.4.1 TMJ DISORDER AND TINNITUS ON BOTH SIDES

Diver, male, 23 years old, training for the PADI Open Water licence during holidays in Asia, did some freediving afterwards. He was a very precise and controlling person and when coming home he graduated from university. His first job was already scheduled with an international company, demanding long working days.

Medical History

The diver experienced tinnitus after the Open Water training. Learning new techniques felt exciting to him and he also felt pressure through wanting to do things well. There was no barotrauma. He was aware of clenching the TMJ when concentrating and remembered that he did bite at the regulator while diving. Stiffness in the TMJ was visible when talking (limited mouth opening). The first sound in his ears was an echo during freediving which developed into a whizzing sound and occasionally a high bleep. Sometimes the tinnitus was not present for a short time after waking in the morning. When swallowing, clicking in the ears occurred. He had manual therapy of the high cervical spine, which had aggravated the tinnitus.

On a scale with 100 per cent standing for *unbearable complaints* and 0 per cent for *no sound* he rated the tinnitus as 70 per cent.

Chinese Medicine Diagnosis
Liver-Qi stagnation.

Treatment
LI-4 Hegu, **LIV-3** Taichong, **PC-6** Neiguan, **SP-6** Sanyinjiao, **ST-36** Zusanli, **M-HN-3** Yintang, **GB-2** Tinghui, **TB-17** Yifeng, **ST-6** Jiache, YNSA Ear and TMJ Points both sides, Ear Point: Shenmen.

Result
In three treatments the tinnitus diminished almost completely. We stopped the treatment because he was starting his demanding job. Six months after the treatments I contacted him and he was doing well. In general the tinnitus was hardly noticeable any more, and if he did have a downturn caused by stress he experienced a maximum of 25 per cent in intensity. If the tinnitus became annoying he was able to reduce it through meditation.

2 External Injury
Due to the injury there is Qi and Xue stagnation in the TMJ. The injury can be a trauma locally in the TMJ or high cervical spine, which affects the TMJ.

● Clinical Signs and Symptoms

- Stiffness in TMJ, decreased range of motion (difficulties opening the mouth), shifting, snapping/clicking in the TMJ
- Tension in the jaw muscles, involuntary rhythmic contractions of jaw-closing muscles (*chattering teeth*)
- Pain in the TMJ, which is aggravated by talking, chewing (pain might be described as ear pain)
- Otic fullness, possibly tinnitus
- Headache
- Stiffness of the neck.

Pulse: Wiry (*Xian*) or Choppy (*Se*).

Tongue: No signs (in the initial stage), dark or purple (or with purple stasis spots).

TEMPOROMANDIBULAR JOINT DISORDERS

- **Treatment Principle**
    - Promote the circulation of Qi and Xue.
    - Benefit the TMJ.

- **Acupuncture Points (select from)**

    LI-4 Hegu, **LIV-3** Taichong, **BL-17** Geshu, **SP-10** Xuehai, **GB-34** Yanglingquan, **ST-6** Jiache, **ST-7** Xiaguan, **GB-2** Tinghui, **SI-19** Tinggong, **SI-17** Tianrong, **GB-20** Fengchi, **GB-21** Jianjing, **ST-44** Neiting, Ashi Points, **M-HN-9** Taiyang, YNSA TMJ and Ear Points, Ear Point: TMJ.

- **Explanation**

    - **LI-4–LIV-3** combination promotes the free flow of Qi and Xue (pain, rigidity and contraction of the muscles).
    - **BL-17** and **SP-10** move Xue.
    - **GB-34** is a distal point that benefits the sinews and joints.
    - **ST-6**, **ST-7**, **GB-2**, **SI-19** and **SI-17** benefit the TMJ. **ST-6** improves the range of motion in the TMJ and alleviates tension or spasm in the masseter muscle. **ST-7**, **GB-2**, **SI-19** and **SI-17** also benefit the ears (tinnitus).
    - **GB-20** in the case of occipital headache or stiffness of the neck.
    - **GB-21** can be used if there is a Trigger Point found at this point (see 'Clinical Notes' in Section 1.12.4B).
    - **ST-44** is an effective distal point to treat the TMJ. Especially good to use when the TMJ itself is too sensitive to needle.
    - Ashi Points (including Trigger Points) relieve pain and muscle tension.
    - Taiyang relaxes the temporalis muscle.
    - YNSA TMJ Point benefits the TMJ in general. If there is tinnitus due to tension in the TMJ region you can add the YNSA Ear Point.
    - Ear Point: TMJ benefits the TMJ in general.
    - Moxa can be used around the TMJ and masseter muscle to improve the circulation of Qi and Xue. Apply gently and at a safe distance from skin and hair.

3 Wind-Cold

This pattern is caused by an invasion of Wind-Cold such as in climate-controlled environments.

● Clinical Signs and Symptoms

- Pain in the TMJ, which is aggravated by talking, chewing (pain might be described as ear pain)
- Stiffness, decreased range of motion
- Tension in the masseter and/or temporalis muscles
- Otic fullness, possibly tinnitus
- Headache
- Stiffness of the neck
- General body ache
- Slight fever
- Chills
- No sweating
- Aversion to cold.

Pulse: Floating (*Fu*) and Wiry (*Xian*).

Tongue: Normal (in the initial stage) or with thin white coating.

● Treatment Principle

- Expel Wind-Cold.
- Benefit the TMJ and warm the muscles.

● Acupuncture Points (select from)

LI-4 Hegu, **TB-5** Waiguan, **ST-6** Jiache, **ST-7** Xiaguan, **GB-2** Tinghui, **GB-20** Fengchi, **GB-21** Jianjing, Ashi Points, **M-HN-9** Taiyang, YNSA TMJ and Ear Points, Ear Point: TMJ.

● Explanation

- **LI-4** and **TB-5** eliminate Wind-Cold. **LI-4** alleviates pain and relieves rigidity of the muscles.
- **ST-6**, **ST-7** and **GB-2** expel Wind and benefit the TMJ. Use **ST-6** when there is tension in the masseter muscle. **ST-7** and **GB-2** benefit the ears.

- **GB-20** expels Wind. Use in the case of occipital headache, stiffness of the neck or blocked ears.

- **GB-21** can be used if there is a Trigger Point found at this point (see 'Clinical Notes' in Section 1.12.4B).

- Ashi Points (including Trigger Points) relieve pain and muscle tension.

- Taiyang relaxes the temporalis muscle.

- YNSA TMJ and Ear Points benefit the TMJ and ear.

- Ear Point: TMJ benefits the TMJ in general.

- Moxa can be used around the TMJ and masseter muscle to expel the Cold and warm the muscles. Apply gently and at a safe distance from skin and hair.

4 Liver-Xue Stasis

Liver-Xue stasis can be caused by chronic Liver-Qi stagnation or Liver-Xue deficiency but also by toxification and obstruction by parasites. Liver-Xue stasis can produce high tension in and contractions of the jaw muscles.

Parasites in the liver can be, for example, roundworms or flatworms that enter the mouth in contaminated water or raw or undercooked meat or fish. People also can become infected (and infect other people as well) if they don't wash their hands after visiting the lavatory. The release of toxins by the parasites in the human body might cause restlessness and anxiety during sleep, triggering bruxism.

● Clinical Signs and Symptoms

- Stiffness in the TMJ, decreased range of motion (difficulties opening the mouth), shifting, snapping/clicking in the TMJ

- Tension in the jaw muscles, cramps, rhythmic contractions of jaw-closing muscles (*tipping teeth*)

- Pain in the TMJ, which is aggravated by talking or chewing (pain might be described as ear pain)

- Otic fullness, possibly tinnitus

- Headache.

Pulse: Wiry (*Xian*) or Choppy (*Se*).

Tongue: Purple (sides or whole tongue) or with purple stasis spots.

- **Treatment Principle**
    - Spread Liver-Qi and Liver-Xue.
    - Benefit the TMJ.

- **Acupuncture Points** (select from)
  LI-4 Hegu, **LIV-3** Taichong, **PC-6** Neiguan, **SP-10** Xuehai, **LIV-8** Ququan, **ST-6** Jiache, **ST-7** Xiaguan, **GB-2** Tinghui, **SI-19** Tinggong, **SI-17** Tianrong, **GB-20** Fengchi, **GB-21** Jianjing, **GB-34** Yanglingquan, **ST-44** Neiting, Ashi Points, **M-HN-9** Taiyang, YNSA TMJ and Ear Points, Ear Points: Shenmen and TMJ, Wrist Point 4.

- **Explanation**
    - **LI-4–LIV-3** combination and **PC-6** spread Liver-Qi. **LI-4** and **LIV-3** combination promotes the circulation of Xue as well.
    - **SP-10** moves Xue.
    - **LIV-8** nourishes Liver-Xue, which is necessary when there is long-term Xue stasis.
    - **ST-6**, **ST-7**, **GB-2**, **SI-19** and **SI-17** benefit the TMJ (pain, muscle tension, dislocation). **ST-6** improves the range of motion in the TMJ and alleviates tension or spasm in the masseter muscle. **ST-7**, **GB-2**, **SI-19** and **SI-17** also benefit the ears (where there is tinnitus due to the TMJ disorder).
    - **GB-20** in the case of occipital headache or stiffness of the neck.
    - **GB-21** can be used if there is a Trigger Point found at this point (see 'Clinical Notes' in Section 1.12.4B).
    - **GB-34** is a distal point that benefits the sinews and joints.
    - **ST-44** is an effective distal point to treat the TMJ. Especially good to use when the TMJ itself is too sensitive to needle.
    - Ashi Points (including Trigger Points) relieve pain and muscle tension.
    - Taiyang relaxes the temporalis muscle.
    - YNSA TMJ Point benefits the TMJ in general. If there is tinnitus due to tension in the TMJ region you can add the YNSA Ear Point.
    - Ear Points: Shenmen calms the Shen and the TMJ Point benefits the TMJ in general.

- Wrist Point 4 benefits the TMJ.
- Moxa can be used around the TMJ and masseter muscle to improve the circulation of Qi and Xue. Apply gently and at a safe distance from skin and hair.

● Clinical Notes

- To treat parasites thoroughly you will have to prescribe herbal medication as well. The combination of wormwood, black walnut and cloves is very effective.

● Food

Pumpkin seeds, coconut, turmeric, hot peppers, garlic, onions. No sugar or cow's milk as they activate the parasites; no coffee or alcohol while detoxing as they overload the intestines and liver. A good *detox soup*, which supports the liver, is made of courgettes, celery, green beans and parsley (cooked in water until they are done and then briefly blended); take a cup of this green soup twice a day.[25]

5 Spleen-Qi Deficiency

Excessive rumination, using too much sugar, a poor diet or antibiotics can deplete the Spleen. The Spleen nourishes the muscles and deficiency can lead to muscle problems in the TMJ. Deficiency of Spleen-Qi can lead to Xue deficiency as the Spleen makes Gu Qi, which is the origin of Xue. Deficiency of Xue can result in Liver-Xue deficiency. The Liver nourishes the sinews and malnourishment can lead to muscle cramps/contractions.

● Clinical Signs and Symptoms

- Borborygmus, distension of the belly
- Tiredness in the morning
- Bruising easily (hematoma)
- Heaviness/puffiness of the body
- TMJ signs and symptoms (pain (often described as ear pain), stiffness, muscle tension, tinnitus etc.).

Pulse: Deficient (*Xu*) or Weak (*Ruo*).

Tongue: Toothmarks, pale, swollen.

---

25 Recipe from Bieler, H.G., *Food Is Your Best Medicine*, Ballantine Books, New York, 2010.

- **Treatment Principle**
    - Tonify Spleen-Qi.
    - Benefit the TMJ.

- **Acupuncture Points (select from)**
  SP-6 Sanyinjiao, **SP-4** Gongsun, **SP-3** Taibai, **BL-20** Pishu, **ST-36** Zusanli, **SP-10** Xuehai, **ST-6** Jiache, **ST-7** Xiaguan, **GB-2** Tinghui, **SI-19** Tinggong, **GB-20** Fengchi, **GB-21** Jianjing, **GB-34** Yanglingquan, Ashi Points, **M-HN-9** Taiyang, YNSA TMJ and Ear Points, Ear Point: TMJ.

- **Explanation**
    - **SP-6**, **SP-4**, **SP-3** and **BL-20** tonify Spleen-Qi.
    - **ST-36** fortifies the Spleen and tonifies Qi in general.
    - **SP-10** invigorates Xue.
    - **ST-6**, **ST-7**, **GB-2** and **SI-19** benefit the TMJ. Use **ST-6** when there is tension in the masseter muscle. **ST-7**, **GB-2** and **SI-19** also benefit the ears.
    - **GB-20** in the case of occipital headache or stiffness of the neck.
    - **GB-21** can be used if there is a Trigger Point found at this point (see 'Clinical Notes' in Section 1.12.4B).
    - **GB-34** is a distal point that benefits the sinews and joints.
    - Ashi Points (including Trigger Points) relieve pain and muscle tension.
    - Taiyang relaxes the temporalis muscle.
    - YNSA TMJ and Ear Points benefit the TMJ and Ear.
    - Ear Point: TMJ benefits the TMJ in general.

- **Food**
  Reduce sugar as much as possible. No cold foods. Cooked foods, chickpeas and ginseng are good to support the Spleen-Qi.

TEMPOROMANDIBULAR JOINT DISORDERS

Table 2.4.1 Important points for TMJ disorders

Local points	Distal points	Special points
ST-6 Jiache	LI-4 Hegu	Ear Point: TMJ
ST-7 Xiaguan	LIV-3 Taichong	YNSA TMJ Point
SI-19 Tinggong	GB-21 Jianjing	Wrist Point 4
GB-2 Tinghui	ST-44 Neiting	
TB-17 Yifeng	ST-36 Zusanli	
SI-17 Tianrong	GB-34 Yanglingquan	
Ashi Points (including Trigger Points)	GB-42 Diwuhui	

● YNSA TMJ Point

The TMJ Point can be used for all TMJ disorders and given my experience this point is especially helpful in the case of bruxism. The YNSA TMJ Point is *not* described by Dr Toshikatsu Yamamoto but by Dr Richard A. Feely who has studied with Dr Yamamoto.[26]

Location: Approximately midway between the YNSA Mouth and Ear Points located at the forehead (palpate from the Mouth Point upwards and laterally about one-half to two-thirds of the way to the Ear Point (see Figure 1.7.3).

● Massage

Besides acupuncture the patient can be treated with physiotherapy and do some self-massages of the jaw muscles to support the treatment. These self-massage techniques must be instructed clearly by the physiotherapist because it is important that they are performed well.

⬇ Advice for the Diver

- When you buy a regulator go to a professional dive store where they can check that the regulator fits well in your mouth before you buy it.

- Don't clamp unnecessarily. When there is some current you will have to clamp a little else you might lose your regulator.

- Be as relaxed as you can when diving. Diminish feelings of anxiety/fear by making clear arrangements with your buddy about how deep you will go, maximum dive time and so on. If you are easily stressed it is better not to drink coffee or cola before your dive.

---

26 Feely, R.A., *Yamamoto New Scalp Acupuncture*, Thieme, New York, 2006.

- If you have bruxism, you might visit a dentist-gnathologist or an oral surgeon and let him or her make a night splint for you to protect your teeth and TMJ. Work with an orofacial physical therapist on relaxing and correcting the position of the TMJ. There are some massage techniques the therapist can teach you to support the relaxation of the jaw muscles. It is important to perform them well.

  You also can use a small massager, which you can use with some oil on the skin to relax the jaw muscles from the outside of the face. The physiotherapist can teach you how to use this massager, but using your own hands is the most easy and practical way and gives immediate feedback about the muscle tension.

  Treating your own jaw muscles should be done very carefully because pressing too hard will give more tension and also might irritate parts of the trigeminal nerve laying quite close to the TMJ.

Try to find the reason why you have bruxism. Some people clench for a big part of the day because they are very focused on what they are doing. Other people might be very perfectionistic and give themselves so much pressure to work well that the tension of the jaw increases incredibly.

Also, having parasites in the intestines, which may have been picked up while travelling, can cause jaw clenching or bruxism. Parasites can spread in the body and hide in the liver, and this organ has an energetic connection with the jaw. Also the toxins from the parasites may result in being tense while sleeping and trigger bruxism.

If your stools change after a diving holiday please visit a physician and ask him or her to check your blood and stools. Parasites can be very difficult to find because the eggs don't emerge with the stools every day (sometimes only once in three weeks). A triple faeces test is advised because the stools will be examined over three days, which makes the chance of finding parasites a little higher. A negative test does not imply that the person is not infected. The test can be *false negative*.

Because being underwater can be like meditation for lots of divers it also can be a very good way to relax and get rid of some jaw muscle tension. The mouthpiece of the regulator can cause a little extra space in the TMJ, which may even contribute to less clenching and more relaxing in the TMJ.

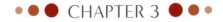

CHAPTER 3

SEASICKNESS
晕动病

3.1 INTRODUCTION

There are amazing day boat trips and live-a-boards (where you stay on a boat for several days). On these trips you can discover some exciting diving spots near and far. Seasickness can disturb a lot of pleasure on a diving holiday. Being sick on a boat is a horrible feeling and might not be necessary. Some acupuncture treatments before a diving holiday can add to a much more comfortable trip. Acupuncture can reduce stress and might take away a big trigger for being seasick.

It is well known by divers that there is usually a certain tension early in the morning on a diving boat. Divers are focused on preparing their equipment, checking air and their underwater cameras. They are thinking of the dives that are coming, and the first planned dive is discussed together with the Divemaster by means of a *briefing*. They will be thinking about specific features of the dive such as the maximum depth they will go, the maximum bottom time, where they hope they will be able to spot some beautiful corals or fish, at which spot they may use a reef hook to be able to watch sharks pass by. A reef hook enables the diver to stay at a place with a strong current without using lots of air in a short time by swimming against the current, or drifting away in a couple of seconds from a very interesting site. The unknown circumstances may give stress to the diver. Diving is a very accurate and alert activity and optimal concentration is requisite. The sharp focus can result in some tension before or during the dive.

Western Medicine
Definition and Aetiology

Seasickness or motion sickness means stimulation of the vestibular organ as a result of movements without visual observation of the movements. The eyes follow the ongoing movements of the boat (the body makes the same movements as the boat) whereby they perceive *standstill*. This does not match with the movements registered by the vestibular organ and the contradictory impulses confuse the brain, with nausea as a consequence.

The semicircular canals in the vestibular organ register turning movements (*rotational acceleration*). The two otolith organs, responsible for registering *linear acceleration*, include the utricule (*horizontal acceleration*: left–right and forward–backward) and the saccule (*vertical acceleration*: up–down). Normally motion sickness (boat, car, airplane, bus) stops when the movements cease.

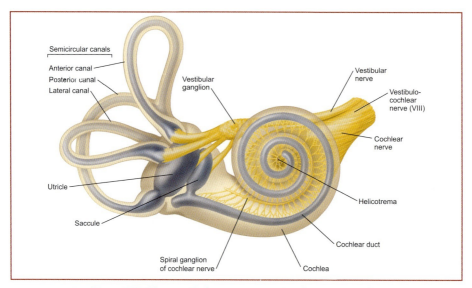

Figure 3.1.1 The vestibular organ contains the semicircular canals and the otolith organs: the utricle and saccule

BOX 3.1.1 SEASICKNESS AND NAUSEA

Hippocrates was the first physician to describe seasickness: 'Sailing on the sea proves that motion disorders the body.' The word 'nausea' derives from the Greek word *naus*, which means *ship*.

Clinical Signs and Symptoms

- Nausea
- Vomiting
- Increased salivation
- Pale skin
- Cold sweats
- Dizziness

- Headache
- Palpitations
- Tiredness.

Treatment
Motion sickness medication blocks the stimulation of the vomiting centre. This reduces the nausea and retching.

Side-effects of motion sickness medication are drowsiness, reduced responsiveness and coordination capacity, and sometimes a dry mouth. Driving a car or performing risky activities after taking motion sickness medication is discouraged. Having a dry mouth when diving is very uncomfortable because the air from the regulator is dry already and the mouth can become very dry in the later part of the dive, which makes swallowing less easy.

Antiemetics (medication against vomiting and nausea) include cinnarizine, which is sedating and can trigger nitrogen narcosis. Cyclizine is the most safe.

Scopolamine patches, which you can place behind the ear, are safe and can be used on the boat.

Chinese Medicine
Diagnosis and Aetiology
The pattern I see in my practice, when treating divers with seasickness, is *Liver-Qi attacking the Stomach* due to feelings of stress. The Stomach-Qi fails to descend due to the stagnation of Liver-Qi. In long-term Liver-Qi stagnation Heat or Phlegm can develop.

Frequently there is an underlying fear or anxiety, which is a risk factor for seasickness because it causes stress.

Diving might be quite stressful, such as if on a boat trip on a wild bumpy sea, which makes it difficult to jump as a group into the water, and the movements of the boat will already be triggering the vestibular organ. In such a situation divers usually have to jump into the water with a jacket that is *not* filled with air from the tank. This way the divers will sink directly under the water surface and will not float at the surface waiting for the other divers before sinking down, because in that situation all the divers would drift away from each other due to the big waves and the current.

Divers might also worry about how the current will be under water or if there might even be a *washing machine*; this is a strong circling water current, and the only way to get out of it is to ascend slowly to the water surface.

It's important to know that cool divers will not find it easy to tell you they ever experience fear or stress under water.

- ● Clinical Signs and Symptoms
  Pulse: Wiry (*Xian*).

  Tongue: No signs or dark (darkish sides or whole tongue).

- ● Treatment Principle
    - Spread Liver-Qi.
    - Soothe the Stomach.
    - Calm the vestibular organ and Shen.

- ● Acupuncture Points (select from)

  PC-6 Neiguan, **LI-4** Hegu, **LIV-3** Taichong, **ST-25** Tianshu, **ST-44** Neiting, **HT-7** Shenmen.

  Ear Points for Seasickness according to Terry Oleson's *Auriculotherapy Manual*: Inner Ear.C, Inner Ear.E, Stomach, Occiput, Point Zero, Shenmen, Lesser Occipital Nerve, Master Oscillation.[1]

- ● Explanation
    - **PC-6** spreads Liver-Qi, soothes the Stomach (nausea, vomiting) and calms the Shen (fear) and vestibular organ.
    - **LI-4–LIV-3** combination spreads Liver-Qi and calms the Shen.
    - **ST-25** and **ST-44** soothe the Stomach and calm the Shen.
    - **HT-7** calms the Shen.
    - Ear Points: Inner Ear.C, Inner Ear.E, Stomach, Occiput, Point Zero, Shenmen, Lesser Occipital Nerve and Master Oscillation.
        - Select a maximum of five Ear Points and use semi-permanent auricular needles when a diver goes on holiday. The needles can be retained during travel/flight to the destination but should be removed at least one day before diving so the skin can heal/close. *Don't* let the diver go under water with semi-permanent needles in because bacteria may come into contact with the skin under the plaster that covers the needles and cause an infection.

- ● Clinical Notes
    - **PC-6** is *the most pivotal point* to influence the vestibular organ and to diminish nausea. Research shows that 'clinical efficacy of **PC-6** may be mediated

---

1   Oleson, T., *Auriculotherapy Manual*, third edition, Churchill Livingstone, Elsevier, London, 2005.

by the cerebellar vestibular neuromatrix' when stimulated by acupuncture (Yoo *et al.* 2004[2]). This point also has been 'identified as a potentially effective method of reducing PONV' (postoperative nausea and vomiting).[3]

- In practice there are people who experience positive effects from a *wrist bandage* that gives pressure at **PC-6** to relieve motion sickness, but there is no scientific evidence for their use in seasickness. I would recommend trying them anyway.

- When a diver has a lot of stress you can instruct him or her to perform some acupressure on **HT-7** and **PC-6** just before the dive or diving day.

- In the case of Liver-Fire add **LIV-2** Xingjian; use **ST-40** Fenglong combined with **ST-36** Zusanli and/or **SP-6** Sanyinjiao when there is Phlegm.

BOX 3.1.2 GINGER

Research from Lien *et al.* (2003) about the 'Effects of ginger on motion sickness and gastric slow-wave dysrhythmias induced by circular vection' resulted in the following conclusion: 'Ginger effectively reduces nausea, tachygastric activity, and vasopressin release induced by circular vection. In this manner, ginger may act as a novel agent in the prevention and treatment of motion sickness.'[4]

CASE STUDY 3.1.1 MOTION SICKNESS

Diver (36 years, female) with motion sickness.

Medical History
Experiencing seasickness alongside motion sickness when reading something in a car. Having a very busy job with deadlines and long working days.

Chinese Medicine Diagnosis
There was stagnation of Liver-Qi suppressing the Stomach besides deficiency of Spleen-Qi and Kidney-Yin.

---

2   Yoo, S.S., Teh, E.K., Blinder, R.A. and Jolesz, F.A., 'Modulation of cerebellar activities by acupuncture stimulation: Evidence from fMRI study', *NeuroImage* (2004) 22, 2, 932–940 (Abstract), www.ncbi.nlm.nih.gov/pubmed/15193624 (accessed 14 September 2017).

3   Nunley, C., Wakim, J. and Guin, C.J., 'The effects of stimulation of acupressure point p6 on postoperative nausea and vomiting: a review of literature', *Journal of PeriAnesthesia Nursing* (2008) 23, 4, 247–261 (Abstract), www.ncbi.nlm.nih.gov/pubmed/18657760 (accessed 14 September 2017).

4   Lien, H.C., Sun, W.M., Chen, Y.H., Kim, H. Hasler, W. and Owyang, C., 'Effects of ginger on motion sickness and gastric slow-wave dysrhythmias induced by circular vection', *American Journal of Physiology: Gastrointestinal and Liver Physiology* (2003) 284, 3, G481–G489 (Abstract), www.ncbi.nlm.nih.gov/pubmed/12576305 (accessed 14 September 2017).

Treatment
LI-4 Hegu, **LIV-3** Taichong, **PC-6** Neiguan, **SP-6** Sanyinjiao, **ST-25** Tianshu, **ST-36** Zusanli, **ST-44** Neiting, **KI-3** Taixi, **KI-6** Zhaohai, **M-HN-3** Yintang, Ear Points: Shenmen and Stomach. Advice: Fresh ginger tea to soothe the stomach.

Result
I gave six treatments during four months and the complaints were solved. She went to Asia for an adventurous holiday, made a boat trip and travelled by bus along very bumpy roads without having any problems.

Advice for the Diver

- Wear a wristband against seasickness on the boat, which gives acupressure on **PC-6** Neiguan.

- Add some slices of fresh ginger in your tea while having breakfast and in the evening to prevent motion sickness. After vomiting as a result of seasickness, fresh ginger tea will soothe your stomach so you will feel better soon.

- Do not use alcohol, oily or spicy foods before diving or the day before.

- Don't have heavy meals before diving, but likewise don't dive with an empty stomach. A light meal is advised.

- Take care that you have enough fresh air. When you are on a live-a-board or day boat trip it's better to stay on deck instead of being inside the boat.

- When you are on a live-a-board ask for a bedroom on the upper deck and/or at the front of the boat.

- Don't smoke.

- When possible rest your head and close your eyes so the vestibular organ might get less irritated.

- When you have vomited, take care to get enough liquids because the body can be dehydrated. When dehydrated you have more risk of decompression illness on the next dive.

●●● CHAPTER 4 ●●●

DECOMPRESSION ILLNESS
减压病

4.1 THE ONSET OF DECOMPRESSION ILLNESS
减压病的发生

Western Medicine

Decompression illness (DI) is one of the first disorders people think of when talking about diving medical problems, although they do not exactly know what it is. I have added basic information about it in this book to extend the knowledge about diving medicine in general and also to make clear that, for example, an ENT disorder like tinnitus can be seen as a sign of decompression illness as well. Acupuncture might help promote the general condition of the diver, which can contribute to preventing decompression illness. Of course it is of indisputable importance to follow all diving rules relating to the ambient pressure, the ascent rate and the release of nitrogen.

Decompression illness and drowning under and above the water surface are the most common diving accidents. They often occur through panic resulting from overconfidence. People can take on too much risk when they are in a holiday mood and think everything is possible. They dive deeper than they should, omit their safety stops or become panicked when they think they have lost their buddy. Either way: they don't think clearly any more and might ascend too fast.

Accidents under water like myocardial infarction are mostly accidents which would happen above the water surface as well and are not directly related to diving (except that in the beginning of the dive the blood pressure is higher). People might get myocardial infarction under water because of not being trained for the situation.

It's important to have knowledge about decompression illness when treating divers. The relation between health and decompression illness is a crucial factor. You can *not* treat decompression illness itself with acupuncture because the diver has to be treated in a decompression room and must be provided with 100 per cent oxygen. But when you know about the causes of decompression illness your acupuncture treatment might help prevent it. Acupuncture can support the general condition, reduce stress and tiredness and improve the blood circulation, all very important factors when reducing the risk of decompression illness.

When a diver descends the body assimilates more nitrogen due to the increased pressure of the ambient surrounding (*on-gassing*). According to Henry's Law the partial pressure of nitrogen grows proportionally to the diving depth. Tissues that store nitrogen easily are blood and lung tissues. Tissues slow to absorb nitrogen are bones and fat. During the ascent the excess of nitrogen disappears by exhaling (*off-gassing*). The nitrogen needs a certain time to wash out, for which it is important to ascend with a certain speed and to make safety stops. When ascending too quickly the partial pressure of nitrogen in the tissues can't diminish sufficiently (*transcends ambient pressure*). When the overpressure exceeds a certain limit, the nitrogen is released into the body tissues and blood vessels as nitrogen *bubbles*. These bubbles are the cause of the onset of decompression illness. A nitrogen bubble may obstruct a blood vessel, cause a lot of damage in the surrounding of the obstruction and even lead to arterial gas embolism.

Decompression illness also may occur when the diving guidelines are followed well, caused by factors like dehydration, repeated dives and being in poor condition (see 'Risk Factors' below).

To prevent decompression illness there are *decompression tables*, which advise a certain time at a certain depth, a certain time in between several dives combined with safety stops (decompression stops), and an ascent rate of 10 metres per minute. When you dive to 30 metres depth or deeper you are obliged to make a safety stop of three minutes at 5 metres depth before you surface. It's recommended to make a safety stop for every dive less deep than 30 metres as well. When you exceed a depth of 40 metres you must ascend directly and make an urgency stop for eight minutes at 5 metres depth. Making a safety stop is part of the normal procedure of the dive. *During the safety stop the body can eliminate nitrogen before surfacing.*

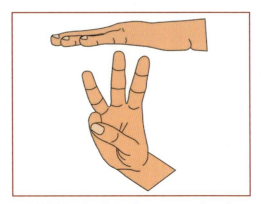

Figure 4.1.1 Diving hand signal to express the safety stop
needed for off-gassing before surfacing
Copyright by Lars Behnke, apporiented.com

Never cough, squeeze, clear or breathe in when ascending because that will make the lung tissues expand! When the elastic limit is exceeded the lung tissues will rupture. Even a small change in pressure can lead to a rupture, especially when taking a deep breath before ascending. *During the ascent you need to exhale so the lungs will not expand due to the decrease in ambient pressure.* Even when ascending from only 1.3 metres depth it is possible to damage the lungs due to the big volume change, and this can lead to mediastinal emphysema, neck emphysema, pneumothorax and arterial gas embolism. Arterial gas embolism (AGE) is the number-one of causes of death when there is pathology.

People mostly ascend too quickly:

- when there is fear or panic
- during an emergency ascent
- as a result of ignorance of the laws of physics that relate to diving
- due to bad dive instruction or poor supervision.

In 50 per cent of DI cases the clinical signs and symptoms manifest themselves within one hour after the ascent, in 90 per cent after six hours. In the case of AGE due to ruptured alveoli the clinical signs and symptoms usually occur within 15 minutes after the ascent and often manifest themselves when reaching the water surface.[1]

Risk Factors

- Ascending too quickly, which gives a pressure change that is too rapid. The sudden overpressure causes the nitrogen gas to release nitrogen bubbles.

- Dehydration leads to less circulating blood volume and blood that gets sticky (off-gassing is more difficult).

- Being in poor condition is a contributory factor because the blood circulation in the tissues is diminished.

- Repeated dives (the body stores nitrogen from previous dives).

- Not enough sleep, tiredness.

- Increasing age. The blood circulation is less good, the blood vessels are poorer quality and general condition becomes poorer.

---

1 Brandt Corstius, J.J., Dermout, S.M. and Feenstra, L., *Duikgeneeskunde, Theorie en Praktijk*, second edition, Elsevier, Amsterdam, 2007.

- Temperature. Cold water leads to vasoconstriction. Ascending to the warmer water levels gives vasodilation, which triggers a release of gas bubbles, as does too rapid warming after the dive (sun, hot shower).

- Alcohol dehydrates the body and reduces sound judgement. For example, nitrogen narcosis may not be recognized.

- Patent foramen ovale (PFO): see Section 1.4 and Figure 1.4.2.

- *Obesity*: at the end of the diving holiday there will be more nitrogen stored in the fat tissues, which release it slowly. If overweight, it is necessary to stop diving one extra day before flying home. This means 48 hours of no diving before flying, as the rule normally is to stop diving 24 hours before flying.

- Hormonal influences might result in more chance of decompression illness during the second half of a woman's cycle due to fluid retention and tissue swelling and less ability to release nitrogen. DAN® (Divers Alert Network)[2] says it might be advisable to dive more conservatively when having PMS (premenstrual syndrome) and during menstruation, especially for women who use oral contraceptives. *Conservative diving* means fewer, shorter and shallower dives and longer safety stops.

- Physical effort such as during drift diving or heavy exercise after the dive may trigger decompression illness. Swimming against the current is quite strenuous and feels uncomfortable quickly in general, and puts increased pressure of the pulmonary arteries and capillaries.

Subdivisions of Decompression Illness[3]

Type I Skin and Joints

- Clinical signs and symptoms: skin
    - itching, burning sensation
    - cutis marmorata
    - exanthema, pain in skin and subcutis.

- Clinical signs and symptoms: joints
    - initially dull pain around the joint and later piercing pain

---

2   Uguccioni, D.M., Moon, R. and Taylor, M.B., 'DAN explores fitness and diving issues in women', DAN: Divers Alert Network, www.diversalertnetwork.org/medical/articles/DAN_Explores_Fitness_and_Diving_Issues_for_Women (accessed 13 August 2017).

3   Brandt Corstius, J.J., Dermout, S.M. and Feenstra, L., *Duikgeneeskunde, Theorie en Praktijk*, tweede druk, Elsevier, Amsterdam, 2007.

- pain increases on moving
- severe fatigue of the affected limbs
- eventually redness and swelling around the affected joint.

Type II Central Nervous System, Stomach and Intestines, Spine, Lungs and Heart

- Clinical signs and symptoms: CNS
    - headache (often first sign)
    - visual disorders
    - aphasia
    - agnosia
    - dizziness
    - disorientation
    - speech disorder
    - unconsciousness and death.

- Clinical signs and symptoms: stomach and intestines
    - nausea
    - decreased appetite
    - diarrhoea
    - abdominal cramps
    - eventually vomiting of blood or blood in diarrhoea.

- Clinical signs and symptoms: spine
    - para-/hemiplegia
    - back pain
    - micturition and defecation disorders.

- Clinical signs and symptoms: lungs
    - sudden dyspnoea
    - pain in thorax, especially when breathing deeply
    - coughing
    - rales (clicking, bubbling or rattling sound when breathing)
    - haemoptysis
    - eventually cyanosis, shock, unconsciousness and death.

- Clinical signs and symptoms: heart
    - angina pectoris
    - nausea and vomiting
    - perspiring
    - agony

- pallor
- irregular heartbeat
- eventually cardiac arrest and death.

Type III Arterial Gas Embolism in Combination with Type II DI

- Clinical signs and symptoms
  - pain in breast
  - dyspnoea
  - dizziness
  - tinnitus
  - sensory disorders
  - visual disorders
  - para-/hemiplegia
  - disorientation
  - convulsions
  - unconsciousness
  - respiratory arrest and sudden death
  - cardiac arrest and sudden death.

Treatment

The usual therapy for decompression illness is to give *100 per cent oxygen* and treatment of the diver in a *decompression room*. It is necessary to give 100 per cent oxygen to provide the area around the blood vessel that is obstructed by the nitrogen bubble as much oxygen as possible to prevent damage.

Chinese Medicine

Reducing tiredness, stress and (if overweight) weight, supporting the blood circulation and stopping smoking can contribute to lowering the risk of decompression illness. Therefore acupuncture can be an effective way to treat divers with physical and mental problems. It is supportive to increase the Qi level of the organs and to promote the smooth circulation of Qi and Xue.

I want to stress again that some acupuncture treatments are very useful before going on a diving holiday, especially when people are stressed and/or tired. The better they feel before they go for a long-distance flight the better they might arrive at the diving destination.

As well as being in good condition it's very important to follow all diving rules at any time! An uncontrolled and too rapid emergency ascent in combination with diving too long, too deep and/or making repetitive dives creates a big risk of getting decompression illness. *Of course acupuncture can't prevent decompression illness in the case of such uncontrolled actions!*

● Treatment Principle

- Check pulse, tongue, face and/or abdomen for your diagnosis.

In general:

- Spread Liver-Qi.
- Strengthen the Lung and promote the descending and diffusing of Lung-Qi.
- Strengthen the Spleen, Kidney, Heart.
- Promote the free flow of Qi and Xue.

● Acupuncture Points (select from)

LI-4 Hegu, **LIV-3** Taichong, **PC-6** Neiguan, **LU-7** Lieque, **LU-9** Taiyuan, **BL-13** Feishu, **SP-6** Sanyinjiao, **SP-4** Gongsun, **SP-3** Taibai, **BL-20** Pishu, **ST-36** Zusanli, **KI-3** Taixi, **KI-6** Zhaohai, **CV-4** Guanyuan, **CV-6** Qihai, **GV-4** Mingmen, **BL-23** Shenshu, **HT-7** Shenmen, **BL-15** Xinshu, **SP-10** Xuehai, **BL-40** Weizhong, **BL-17** Geshu, Ear Point: Shenmen.

● Explanation

- **LI-4–LIV-3** combination and **PC-6** spread Liver-Qi. **LI-4–LIV-3** combination promotes the free flow of Qi and Xue.
- **LU-7**, **LU-9** and **BL-13** strengthen the Lung and promote the descending and diffusing of Lung-Qi.
- **SP-6**, **SP-4**, **SP-3** and **BL-20** strengthen the Spleen.
- **ST-36** supports general tonification.
- **KI-3**, **KI-6**, **CV-4**, **CV-6**, **GV-4** and **BL-23** strengthen the Kidney (for their different actions see Table 1.7.5).
- **HT-7** and **BL-15** strengthen the Heart.
- **SP-10**, **BL-40** and **BL-17** move Xue.
- Ear Point: Shenmen supports general relaxation (release of endorphins).

⬇ Advice for the Diver

- Drink enough water during the flight to your diving destination as the air conditioning in the airplane (dry air) dehydrates your body. DAN® Europe advises drinking 240 ml water every hour of the flight time. Drink enough water before and in between the dives to prevent dehydration. DAN® Europe recommends drinking one glass of water every 15–20 minutes.

- Drink coconut water – which you can find at most tropical dive locations – because it is more hydrating than normal water and it contains electrolytes (magnesium, calcium, sodium, potassium and phosphorus).

- Take your time to recover from jetlag and don't jump in the water directly after arriving at your holiday destination. When you have had a long flight it's best to take one day of rest to recover and adapt to the new and – most of the time – tropical surrounding with higher temperatures.

- Put on your diving suit just before going in the water to prevent dehydration when it's warm. When you sweat a lot before the dive you will lose a lot of body fluids.

- Take care to have sufficient sleep during the whole diving holiday.

- In general eat healthy food and don't take too much coffee before diving because that causes dehydration as well. When you dive in tropical regions there are usually bananas, coconuts, mangos and pineapples which provide a lot of vitamins and minerals.

- Adding some vitamins such as vitamin C and minerals such as magnesium and Omega 3 may support your general well-being and/or the blood circulation in the muscles.

- Adjust the thickness of the diving suit to the temperature of the water so you will not unnecessarily lose body warmth. Wear a hood and/or gloves when the water is really cold or when making a night dive. A night dive is usually less deep (often a maximum of 10 m) and when done wisely is in an area the diver has been before so he or she can recognize the surrounding, but the water cools quickly when the sun goes down.

- After the dive have a freshwater shower as soon as possible so you can get rid of the salt crystals, which may dry on the skin and aggravate dehydration.

- Only sit in the sun after a dive for a short time to dry your body; then it is better to look for a comfortable place in the shade and relax before the next dive.

- Protect your body well in cold diving surroundings as low temperatures also can induce decompression illness. Cold water can result in cold diuresis by which the body can dehydrate.

- After diving you need to wait for 24 hours before flying (back home after your holiday or to another location during your diving holiday). The additional nitrogen in the body – due to the diving – needs time to leave the body tissues. In the air cabin there is an artificially low air pressure of about 0.8 ATA. Because of the decreased air pressure there is still a risk for decompression illness as nitrogen bubbles might expand.

CHAPTER 5

DIVING, MEDICATION AND NATURAL STIMULANTS

潜水 药物和天然兴奋剂

5.1 MEDICATION, SIDE-EFFECTS AND CONTRAINDICATIONS FOR DIVING
潜水用药 副作用和禁忌症

Due to the hydrostatic pressure some medication works more strongly or differently than above the water surface. The pressure under water alters the effect of medication due to a change in the *sodium potassium pump*. For example, antihistamines will be much more sedating and blood thinners make the blood more thin than they normally would.

When using medication it is important to have in mind that the underlying condition itself can be a reason not to dive (e.g. bipolar disorder, severe depression, or cardiac arrhythmia combined with poor general condition/being overweight) besides the side-effects of the medication.

Medication can give the following problems under the water surface:

- Systemic effects.

- Tiredness.

- Hallucinations.

- Reverse block when using xylometazoline (e.g. Otrivin®, Nasivin®) for several dives per day. Pseudoephedrine (e.g. Sudafed®) can solve that problem but can trigger cardiac arrhythmia or raise the blood pressure.

- Antibiotics are mostly safe but can give nausea.

- Medication with vomiting as side-effect may not be used under water because vomiting under the water surface might be dangerous. You can vomit in the regulator so that's no problem but you will feel uncomfortable in general.

- Tetracyclines can cause photosensitivity.

- Sedatives and antihistamines might provoke nitrogen narcosis and can affect awareness. Nitrogen narcosis increases the sedating effect. Aerius®, containing desloratadine, has few side-effects.

- Diuretics cause dehydration and hypokalemia.

- Beta-blockers decrease exercise tolerance. They lower the heart rate, the blood pressure and the VO2 max (a person's maximum rate of oxygen consumption), and lung oedema might be an effect. However, diving with beta-blockers is possible in some specific cases and when using a low dosage. *Diving when using beta-blockers if you have high blood pressure is strongly dissuaded!*

- ACE-inhibitors can cause coughing. Test the ACE-inhibitors in a swimming pool. If they cause no problems you can dive with them.

- Digoxines are mostly safe.

- Anticoagulants (e.g. coumarin) and antiplatelets (e.g. aspirin) can be absolute or relative contraindications for diving. They can cause bleeding during or after the dive. Coumarins are absolutely contraindicated when diving. Aspirin is safe to use.

    - *Antiplatelets:* 'less severe bleeding *but* particularly at sites of diving-related stress (ENT), immediate effects (during the dive)'[1]

    - *Anticoagulants:* 'potentially more severe bleeding *but* delayed bleeding (i.e. after the dive)'[2] for example in the spinal cord.

- Antimalarial: Lariam can lead to bradycardia and mental problems, and provoke epileptic seizures.

- Medication often results in dehydration of the body so there is more chance of decompression illness.

- Corticosteroids and nitrofurantoin might increase sensitivity for oxygen toxicity.

---

1   Westerweel, P., 'Medication Used in Internal Medicine and Diving', in N.A.M. Schellart (ed.) *A Comprehensive Textbook of Medication and Diving*, Capita Selecta Duikgeneeskunde Volume 13, Stichting Duik Research, Amsterdam, 2016.

2   Westerweel, P., 'Medication Used in Internal Medicine and Diving', in N.A.M. Schellart (ed.) *A Comprehensive Textbook of Medication and Diving*, Capita Selecta Duikgeneeskunde Volume 13, Stichting Duik Research, Amsterdam, 2016.

- Psychological medication that disinhibits can be very dangerous because the diver might not recognize safety and/or danger clearly, which can result in taking too much risk. Sedating effects can influence the awareness and trigger nitrogen narcosis.

   When taking medication for ADHD, the ADHD itself is a reason to declare someone unfit to dive because ADHD involves focusing problems. A good focus is very important when diving.

- Antidepressants might cause convulsions and nitrogen narcosis. SSRIs (selective serotonin reuptake inhibitors) can cause disinhibition and a higher risk of bleeding.

- Antiemetics: cinnarizin is sedating and can trigger nitrogen narcosis. Scopolamine patches are safe.

Clinical Notes

- When using/needing *any* medication it is necessary to discuss the disorder and possible side-effects of the medication with a diving physician to be clear if there are any consequences for diving.

5.2 DIVING AND MIGRAINE
潜水和偏头痛

When you feel well, diving is a spectacular experience. Having a migraine when you want to start a dive is a contraindication for diving because you don't feel good, you might vomit or experience vision problems, you can't concentrate and the cold water might aggravate the complaint. Also some migraine medication does not allow a diver to go under water and the diver is probably not thinking of diving at all. These are all reasons to find a way to eliminate migraines and make diving possible.

Western Medicine
Definition and Aetiology

Migraine is a neurovascular disorder, characterized by recurrent episodic attacks of headache, usually throbbing and unilateral and often accompanied by an aura (visual problems – light flashes, stains, asterisks or visual field loss – and tingling or deaf feeling arm, leg or face) and vomiting.

   The cause of the onset of migraine is still unclear despite lots of research. The aura is almost surely caused by *cortical spreading depression (CSD)*: hyperactivity of certain cells in the brain stem followed by almost complete extinction. CSD provokes an increased activity of the trigemino vascular system resulting in vasodilatation of blood vessels in the meninges. The dilatation causes pressure on the nerve endings around the blood vessels resulting in pain and inflammation around the blood vessels.

Migraine patients have an increased sensitivity for certain stimuli and often there is a strong familial influence. Triggers of migraine are among other things: stress, muscle tension and facet joint problems in the cervical spine, hormones (birth control pills, menses, menopause), food (irregular/skipped meals, not enough food, coffee, cheese, alcohol (sulphite), monosodium glutamate (E621), aspartame), weather changes, physical exertion and altered sleeping patterns.

Migraine while diving might be triggered by:

- the cold water influencing the temperature of the head and the mucosa of the nose and sinuses
- stress
- spine problems
- clenching the regulator (overstimulation of the TMJ).

When a migraine attack occurs under water the diver must warn his or her buddy directly and end the dive, which implies ascending to the surface and going back to the shore or boat.

A headache that starts under water might be caused by:

- a hood or mask that is too tight
- the cold water influencing the temperature of the head and the mucosa
- a low blood glucose level
- hyperventilation and skip breathing (holding the breath to try to conserve air)
- stress
- clamping on the regulator (overstimulation of the TMJ)
- spine problems
- oxygen toxicity
- nitrogen narcosis.

Treatment

Medication (among others):

- Paracetamol

- NSAIDs
- Triptans (serotonin receptor agonists) like sumatriptan (e.g. Imigran) which constrict the blood vessels in the brain
- Beta-blockers (preventive).

Clinical Notes

- When using sumatriptan, diving is not allowed because of the side-effects, such as dizziness, vertigo, weakness, drowsiness, nausea and vomiting.

Chinese Medicine
Definition and Aetiology

Migraine (Tou Tong) can be divided in Tou Feng (Wind in the head) and Pian Tou Tong (Pain of half of the head) and is mostly caused by disturbed emotions, which lead to Liver-Yang rising and internal Wind, disturbed hormones, certain foods (e.g. coffee, alcohol, hot chillies), sleeping problems, physical exertion and cervical problems.

In general people react very well to acupuncture when suffering from migraines and can get rid of them totally. Migraines have an enormous influence on people because it can be impossible for them to function well in daily life. Going to work might be ruled out and social contacts might be limited. Diving is possible (again) when someone gets rid of the migraine attacks.

Pattern Differentiation
1 Hyperactivity of Liver-Yang

Stress, mental upset, anger, hot food and drinks (alcohol, coffee, hot chillies, peppers) can cause Liver-Qi stagnation, Liver-Fire, consumption of Liver-Yin and in the end Liver-Yang rising.

> **BOX 5.2.1 LONG-TERM DISTURBANCE OF THE LIVER FUNCTION**
>
> Prolonged Liver-Qi stagnation ➔ Liver-Fire ➔ Liver-Yin Deficiency ➔ Liver-Yang Rising

● Clinical Signs and Symptoms

- Headache (frontal, temporal, eye), throbbing or pounding pain

- Blurred vision, red and sore eyes
- Dizziness with distended feeling in the head
- Flushes in the face
- Thirst, bitter taste in the mouth
- Nausea, vomiting
- Photophobia and hyperacusis
- Constipation
- Insomnia
- Irritability
- Restlessness.

Pulse: Wiry (*Xian*) and Rapid (*Shuo*).

Tongue: Red with a thin yellow coating.

● Treatment Principle
 − Spread Liver-Qi.
 − Nourish Liver-Yin.
 − Subdue Liver-Yang.
 − Calm the Shen.

● Acupuncture Points (select from)
LI-4 Hegu, **LIV-3** Taichong, **PC-6** Neiquan, **LIV-2** Xingjian, **LIV-8** Ququan, **SP-6** Sanyinjiao, **GB-20** Fengchi, **GB-8** Shuaigu, **GV-20** Baihui, **GV-24** Shenting, **GV-23** Shangxing, YNSA Basic A Point, **M-HN-3** Yintang, **M-HN-9** Taiyang, Ear Point: Shenmen.

● Explanation
- **LI-4**–**LIV-3** combination and **PC-6** spread Liver-Qi.
- **LIV-2** clears Liver-Fire and spreads Liver-Qi.
- **LIV-8** nourishes Liver-Yin.
- **SP-6** spreads Liver-Qi, harmonizes the Liver and nourishes Yin in general. Good point to support this condition.
- **GB-20**, **GB-8** and **GV-20** subdue Liver-Yang.

- **GV-24** and **GV-23** benefit the head and eyes and calm the Shen. **GV-24** calms the Liver as well. **GV-23** can be used in the case of any fullness or deficiency of the head.

- YNSA Basic A Point alleviates headache/migraine of any origin. You can instruct your patient to do acupressure on this point.

- Yintang relieves frontal headache, Taiyang temporal (one-sided) headache.

- Ear Point: Shenmen calms the Shen.

2 Kidney-Yin Deficiency

Kidney-Yin deficiency can be caused by overwork, excessive sexual activity, loss of Jin Ye and/or Xue and chronic illness.

● Clinical Signs and Symptoms

- Headache with empty feeling in the head
- Dizziness
- Tinnitus
- Blurred vision
- Weakness in the lower back and knees
- Five-palm Heat
- Night sweating.

Pulse: Thready (*Xi*) and Rapid (*Shuo*).

Tongue: Red and dry with a slight, yellow or no coating.

● Treatment Principle

– Nourish Kidney-Yin.

● Acupuncture Points (select from)

KI-3 Taixi, **KI-6** Zhaohai, **CV-4** Guanyuan, **BL-23** Shenshu, **SP-6** Sanyinjiao, **GV-23** Shangxing, YNSA Basic A Point, **M-HN-3** Yintang, **M-HN-9** Taiyang.

● Explanation

- **KI-3**, **KI-6**, **CV-4** and **BL-23** nourish Kidney-Yin.

- **SP-6** nourishes Yin in general. Good point to support this condition.

- **GV-23** benefits the head.

- YNSA Basic A Point alleviates headache/migraine of any origin. You can instruct your patient to do acupressure on this point.

- Yintang relieves frontal headache, Taiyang temporal (one-sided) headache.

Clinical Notes

- In the case of migraine the YNSA Basic A Point (Yin side) is very effective (see Figure 1.7.3 and 'YNSA Basic Points' in Section 6.2). The Basic A Point influences the head, the cervical spine and the areas innervated by the cervical nerves. When I use this point bilaterally the condition decreases enormously in a short time, often totally. The diver can do some massage of the A Points him or herself to support the acupuncture treatment (softly with their fingers to reduce the tension and pain still left at the A Point). When you provide a drawing of the Basic A Points they can be found easily by palpating the inner corner of the eyebrow and from there going straight up into the hairline.

  I love combining the YNSA points with body acupuncture because from my clinical experience I can say the effects are strong and very positive! There are patients who recovered from migraines totally after experiencing them for 8 or 12 years. Usually four to eight acupuncture sessions are sufficient. When possible I send these patients home with a couple of scalp needles still in their head so they can keep them in for about three more hours. This greatly strengthens the effect of the treatment.

Advice for the Diver

- Be careful with cold water diving (even when wearing a hood). The head is very sensitive to extremes of temperature (hot and cold) and changes in temperature. Under water we lose most body heat through the head. The deeper you dive the colder it gets. In non-tropical regions the water is much colder than in tropical seas and oceans, and most of the time you will need to wear a hood to protect your head from cooling.

- Go to a licensed acupuncturist for some acupuncture treatments so you can be cured of those horrible migraine attacks. It is important to visit an acupuncturist who is also a physician or physiotherapist, because Western diagnostics are needed to check, for example, the range of motion of the cerebral spine, to discover if there is a facet joint problem, or a dislocation of a vertebra.

5.3 DIVING AND HYPERTENSION
潜水和高血压
Western Medicine
Definition and Aetiology
This section will deal with the treatment of primary (or essential) hypertension, which means systemic arterial hypertension of unknown cause. Primary hypertension is often family related but also can be caused by multiple factors like stress, smoking, being overweight and not getting enough physical exercise.

Hypertension is divided into:

- a *slightly elevated* blood pressure (systolic blood pressure (SBP) > 140 mmHg)
- a *moderately elevated* blood pressure (SBP > 160 mmHg)
- a *strongly elevated* blood pressure (SBP > 180 mmHg)
- a *very severe* hypertension (SBP > 200 mmHg)

In secondary hypertension there is an underlying condition like kidney disease, or a factor such as overconsumption of liquorice that causes the hypertension.

Treatment
Medication (among other things):

- Beta-blockers
- Diuretics
- Ace-inhibitors
- Angiotensin II blockers
- Calcium blockers
- Vasodilators.

Important lifestyle advice:

- Take daily exercise like walking, cycling, swimming, gardening and focus in general on relaxation.
- Eat healthy food.
- Lose weight if overweight.
- Stop smoking (if applicable).

Clinical Notes

- Diving is strongly discouraged if taking beta-blockers for high blood pressure! To get a patient fit for diving again you can help to normalize the hypertension with acupuncture so no medication is needed any more.

Chinese Medicine
Aetiology

In my practice I mostly see hypertension accompanied by (1) chronic stress because people have busy jobs resulting mainly in problems of the Liver and Kidney, and (2) Phlegm-Damp due to improper diet and disturbed emotions.

Pattern Differentiation
1 Hyperactivity of Liver-Yang

Stress, mental upset, anger, hot food and drinks (alcohol, coffee, hot chillies, peppers) can cause Liver-Qi stagnation, Liver-Fire, consumption of Liver-Yin and in the end Liver-Yang rising (see Box 5.2.1).

Clinical Signs and Symptoms

- Headache aggravated by mental upset (occipital, cranial)
- Dizziness with distended feeling in the head
- Tinnitus
- Bitter taste in the mouth
- Nausea, vomiting
- Constipation
- Flushes in the face
- Blurred vision, red and sore eyes
- Photophobia
- Dream-disturbed sleep
- Irritability

Pulse: Wiry (*Xian*) and Rapid (*Shuo*).

Tongue: Red with yellow coating.

- ● Treatment Principle
    - – Spread Liver-Qi.
    - – Clear Liver-Fire.
    - – Nourish Liver-Yin.
    - – Subdue Liver-Yang.

- ● Acupuncture Points (select from)
  LI-4 Hegu, **LIV-3** Taichong, **PC-6** Neiguan, **LIV-2** Xingjian, **LIV-8** Ququan, **LI-11** Quchi, **GB-20** Fengchi, **GB-8** Shuaigu, **GV-20** Baihui, **SP-6** Sanyinjiao, **GV-24** Shenting, YNSA Basic A Point, **M-HN-3** Yintang, **M-HN-9** Taiyang.

- ● Explanation
    - **LI-4–LIV-3** combination and **PC-6** spread Liver-Qi.
    - **LIV-2** clears Liver-Fire and spreads Liver-Qi.
    - **LIV-8** nourishes Liver-Yin.
    - **LI-11** clears Heat, regulates the circulation of Qi and Xue and is very effective in decreasing high blood pressure.
    - **GB-20**, **GB-8** and **GV-20** subdue Liver-Yang.
    - **SP-6** spreads Liver-Qi, harmonizes the Liver and tonifies Yin in general. Good point to support this condition.
    - **GV-24** benefits the head and eyes and calms the Liver and Shen.
    - YNSA Basic A Point alleviates headache of any origin. You can instruct your patient to do acupressure on this point.
    - Yintang relieves frontal headache, Taiyang temporal (one-sided) headache.

- ● Food[3]
    - Restrict or avoid hot substances, highly saturated fats and oils, cold or refrigerated food.
    - Don't overeat, and prevent turbulent emotions during meals.
    - Focus on vegetables and fruits. Carbohydrates and proteins should be less than half of the diet.

---

3 Maclean, W. and Lyttleton, J., *Clinical Handbook of Internal Medicine*, Volume 2, second printing, University of Western Sydney, Sydney, 2003.

2 Kidney-Yin Deficiency

Kidney-Yin deficiency can be caused by overwork, excessive sexual activity, loss of Jin Ye and/or Xue and chronic illness.

● Clinical Signs and Symptoms

- Headache or dizziness together with an empty feeling in the head
- Tinnitus
- Deafness
- Blurred vision
- Weakness of the lower back and knees
- Dry mouth
- Five-palm Heat
- Night sweating.

Pulse: Thready (*Xi*) and Rapid (*Shuo*).

Tongue: Red and dry with a slight, yellow or no coating.

● Treatment Principle

— Nourish Kidney-Yin.

● Acupuncture Points (select from)

KI-3 Taixi, **KI-6** Zhaohai, **CV-4** Guanyuan, **BL-23** Shenshu, **SP-6** Sanyinjiao, YNSA Basic A Point, **M-HN-3** Yintang, **M-HN-9** Taiyang.

● Explanation

- **KI-3**, **KI-6**, **CV-4** and **BL-23** nourish Kidney-Yin.
- **SP-6** nourishes Yin in general. Good point to support this condition.
- YNSA Basic A Point alleviates headache of any origin. You can instruct your patient to do acupressure on this point.
- Yintang relieves frontal headache, Taiyang temporal headache.

3 Phlegm-Damp

Phlegm-Damp can be caused by overconsumption of greasy and/or fried foods, dairy products and sugar, and can present combined with Spleen-Qi deficiency.

- **Clinical Signs and Symptoms**
    - Distending headache
    - Heavy and foggy head
    - Heavy-feeling body
    - Dizziness
    - Poor appetite
    - Fullness and oppression in chest and epigastrium.

    Pulse: Slippery (*Hua*).

    Tongue: White greasy coating.

- **Treatment Principle**
    - Transform Phlegm/Dampness.

- **Acupuncture Points (select from)**

    ST-40 Fenglong, **CV-12** Zhongwan, **SP-9** Yinlingquan, **LI-11** Quchi, **ST-25** Tianshu, **SP-6** Sanyinjiao, **SP-4** Gongsun, **SP-3** Taibai, **BL-20** Pishu, **ST-36** Zusanli, YNSA Basic A Point, **GB-20** Fengchi, **M-HN-3** Yintang, **M-HN-9** Taiyang.

- **Explanation**
    - **ST-40** and **CV-12** resolve Phlegm and Dampness.
    - **SP-9** transforms Dampness and regulates the Spleen.
    - **LI-11** drains Dampness and lowers the blood pressure.
    - **ST-25** resolves Dampness and eliminates stagnation of Qi, Xue and food in the abdomen.
    - **SP-6**, **SP-4**, **SP-3** and **BL-20** strengthen the Spleen and prevent the formation of Dampness.
    - **ST-36** supports general tonification.
    - YNSA Basic A Point alleviates headache of any origin (you can instruct your patient to do acupressure on this point), **GB-20** when there is a stiff neck as well.
    - Yintang relieves frontal headache and Taiyang temporal headache.

DIVING, MEDICATION AND NATURAL STIMULANTS

● Food
No fried food, no peanuts, no dairy products.

⬇ Advice for the Diver

- You may not dive until the blood pressure is normalized and only if you don't need contraindicated medication any more. Always consult a physician and ask for advice before starting diving (again).
- Release stress (meditation, walking).
- Reduce weight if overweight.
- Stop smoking (if applicable).

5.4 NATURAL STIMULANTS
天然兴奋剂
Diving and Alcohol

In 80 per cent of all drowning accidents among adult male divers alcohol is the cause. Alcohol causes coordination problems, disturbed awareness and dehydration. Alcohol works synergistically with nitrogen under water. It is recommended not to drink alcohol during the diving holiday because of these risk factors. In the case of dehydration the diver is more susceptible to decompression illness.

Diving and Tobacco

Smoking (nicotine) has the following effects:

- Poor-quality blood vessels.
- An increase in blood pressure and acceleration of the heartbeat.
- Contraction of the coronary arteries.[4]
- Stimulation of the central nervous system (noradrenalin, dopamine, serotonin, beta-endorphin) with a 'feeling of well-being and decreased irritability'.[5]

Inhaling tobacco smoke might cause:[6]

---

4   Gaastra, M., 'Welke invloed heeft roken op duiken?', E-letter Duiken, 01-06-2014.
5   Dowd, F.J., Johnson, B.S., Mariotti, A.J., *Pharmacology and Therapeutics for Dentistry*, seventh edition, Elsevier, St Louis, MI. 2017 (p.99).
6   Gaastra M., 'Welke invloed heeft roken op duiken?', E-letter Duiken, 01-06-2014.

- Contractions of the respiratory tract.

- Fewer working cilia.

- Production of mucus, which obstructs the nose and burdens the lungs. It makes the lungs more sensitive to *air trapping*. Air trapping is abnormal air retention in the lungs due to an obstruction. During the ascent there is more chance of an overpressure injury (pneumothorax, pulmonary embolism). In general there will be more difficulties with equalization of the ears and sinuses due to the production of mucus and irritation of the mucosa.

- An increase of carbon monoxide in the blood (5–9%), which can lead to changes on a mental and motoric level. Due to this increase there are fewer red blood cells, which results in less oxygen transportation to the heart and lungs.

Chinese Medicine

Energetically tobacco (nicotine) improves the flow of Liver-Qi. That is why it relaxes people and why they get irritated when trying to stop smoking: the Liver-Qi stagnates.

The problem when being addicted to a particular substance is also that the tongue papillae are used to sensing a specific thing and want it again and again.

Acupuncture can be very supportive, especially affecting the withdrawal symptoms positively after stopping with smoking, such as: dizziness, tiredness, boredom, irritability, cough, nasal congestion or discharge, depression, headache, frustration, insomnia, increased appetite, concentration problems. Always select the points needed for your specific patient as everyone is different.

● Treatment Principle

– Spread Liver-Qi.

– Strengthen the Lung and promote the descending and diffusing of Lung-Qi.

– Calm the Shen.

– Transform Phlegm.

– Open the nose.

● Acupuncture Points (select from)
GB-8 Shuaigu, **LI-4** Hegu, **LI-20** Yingxiang, **LIV-3** Taichong, **PC-6** Neiguan, **LU-7** Lieque, **LU-9** Taiyuan, **HT-7** Shenmen, **ST-40** Fenglong, **ST-44** Neiting.

Ear points according Terry Oleson[7] (select a maximum of five points):

- Primary Points: Nicotine Point, Lung 1, Lung 2, Mouth, Point Zero, Shenmen, Sympathetic Autonomic Point, Brain
- Supplemental: Adrenal Gland C., Aggressivity, Limbic System.

● Explanation

- **GB-8** treats addictions and intoxications (tobacco, alcohol, coffee).[8]
- **LI-4** and **LI-20** benefit the nose (congestion, discharge).
- **LI-4–LIV-3** combination and **PC-6** spread Liver-Qi (in people who smoke to diminish feelings of stress).
- **LU-7** and **LU-9** strengthen the Lung and promote the descending and diffusing of Lung-Qi (cough, mucus).
- **HT-7** calms the Shen (if someone is very restless).
- **ST-40** transforms Phlegm.
- **ST-44** reduces excessive feelings of hunger, which might occur after stopping with smoking.
- Ear Points supporting the treatment: Nicotine Point, Lung 1, Lung 2, Mouth, Point Zero, Shenmen, Sympathetic Autonomic Point, Brain, Adrenal Gland C., Aggressivity and Limbic System.

● Clinical Notes

- It's practical to work with semi-permanent auricular needles so the effect of the treatment is longer-lasting. The effects are the strongest in the first seven hours; after three days the effects decrease considerably. Don't leave the needles in for longer than a week because the skin might become irritated under the plaster and the full effects of the needles will have been achieved.

Diving and Coffee

When people are prone to stress it is advisable to drink no coffee before diving. Caffeine stimulates the production of adrenalin and can lead to tension and restlessness. Not too much coffee is advised anyway when diving because it dehydrates the body by which you are more sensitive for decompression illness.

---

7   Oleson, T., *Auriculotherapy Manual*, third edition, Churchill Livingstone, Elsevier, London, 2005.
8   Boermeester, W., *Tekstboek Acupunctuur, deel I, Punten*, Chinese Medicine Data, Kapellen, 1989.

CHAPTER 6

ADDITIONAL INFORMATION AND ADVICE REGARDING DIVING-RELATED DISORDERS
与潜水有关的附加资料和建议

6.1 INTRODUCTION
In this chapter I will explain the effects of some physical and mental complaints on diving to provide you with an optimal view of a large range of diving medical problems. Pattern differentiation and treatment options are discussed in short and the actions of the needed acupuncture points are explained together in one section. The focus is on seeing the relationship between the complaints and diving.

6.2 NECK AND BACK DISORDERS
颈和腰部疾患

Neck and back disorders are often seen in divers, mostly with professional divers like instructors and Divemasters who frequently have to deal with the weight of the belt on their back, help students to lift their equipment, and carry a lot of diving tanks and other material that is required when preparing a diving instructing day. Bottles need to be filled with compressed air and to be packed in a truck or van. On an average course day usually two dives are made so when there are ten students this means at least 20 diving bottles (and you always need reserve tanks). A standard 12 litre aluminium bottle weights about 15 kilo.

Non-professional divers who have neck and back disorders usually experience them in normal daily life and they want to get rid of them to dive more comfortably.

A weight belt or weight pockets are needed with diving to descend in the water. They are used as a belt above the pelvis or as integrated pockets in the jacket. In an emergency you may need to throw the belt or pockets off and ascend as soon as possible to the water surface – while breathing out to protect the lungs. Integrated weight pockets at the front of the jacket are easier on the back as a weight belt gives pressure at the lumbar region.

Western Medicine

Acupuncture can be done as a main therapy or combined with other medical treatments like physiotherapy and manual therapy. Besides acupuncture it's recommended to combine the treatment with some exercises because for most neck and back disorders it's necessary to give posture corrections and support the functioning of the spine with mobilization, relaxation (massage), muscle strengthening and/or stabilizing exercises.

With all mobilization methods the movements of the vertebrae in relation to each other need to be done three dimensionally because that's the way humans move naturally. When performing passive mobilization techniques it's possible to focus on two vertebrae and move very specifically in between these two bones to regulate the disturbed mobility.

When divers experience neck problems during a dive it is often caused by hyperextension of the cervical spine. This is seen when a diver descends in the water with the head positioned lower than the feet, looking around. While descending it's necessary to keep the head higher than the feet to clear the ears well, and this position prevents developing irritation of the neck.

Lower back problems can occur under water when a heavy weight belt pulls the lower spine in extension, which can result in pain in the lower back and/or radiation into the leg(s). This problem can be solved by using integrated weight pockets in the jacket instead of a weight belt.

Overload and increasing age can lead to a more accelerated process of osteoarthritis, arthritis and disc degeneration.

Osteoarthritis (or arthrosis) is a normal process starting around the age of 20 years – and depending on age some amount of osteoarthritis is seen as normal – but can be aggravated by a mechanical trauma or overload. The symptoms of osteoarthritis are pain and/or stiffness in a joint and *starting problems*. This means the complaints are worst after a time of rest and improve by moving.

Arthritis is a sterile inflammatory reaction of the connective tissues like the capsule of a joint due to mechanical overload or an injury where the skin is not openly damaged.

Disc degeneration is a process that leads to a diminished shock-absorbing function and height loss (the nucleus pulposus loses its moisture).

For diagnosis and treatment of the spine it is important to realize that:[1]

---

1   Marsman, J., Gelevert, B. and Leferink. H., 'Syllabus 2012' handout, Manuele Therapie Marsman (MTM) institute, the Netherlands.

- the human being has a preferred way of moving, and this preference results in opposing movements and restrictions
- the scalp and spine movements are flexion, extension, rotation and lateroflexion
- we can distinguish four combination types of movements:
  - flexion combined with lateroflexion right and rotation left (A)
  - extension combined with lateroflexion right and rotation right (B)
  - flexion combined with lateroflexion left and rotation right (C)
  - extension combined with latcroflexion left and rotation left (D).

The scalp and spine can be divided into the following zones:

- C0–C1–C2 (suboccipital zone)
- C3–C4–C5 (midcervical zone)
- C6–C7–TH1 (cervicothoracic transition)
- TH2–TH6 (high thoracic zone)
- TH7–TH12 (low thoracic zone)
- L1–L5 (lumbar zone)
- Sacrum/coccyx combined with the ilium (SI joint).

The scalp (C0) follows the direction of C1 and they form a unit (C0–C1). When C1 is in flexion, the scalp is in flexion; when C1 is in extension the scalp is in extension. C2 moves in the opposite direction to C1 regarding the flexion/extension and rotation movements.

Another thing to bear in mind when having neck problems is that about 40–45 per cent of the whole rotation happens between C1 and C2, while the total rotation range in the cervical spine is 90 degrees (in a healthy person). Always check the specific level when there are rotation limitations.

Very important for optimal rotation of the head is sufficient extension of the cervicothoracic junction (CTJ). An optimally working CTJ also provides an entire range of motion (180°) in flexion of the arms. People with anteroposition of the head (often due to stress, *wanting to control everything*) have an increased protrusion of C7. This results in insufficient extension of the CTJ and due to that insufficient rotation of the head and a decrease in flexion-elevation of the arms. Mobilizing the CTJ for a couple of minutes before needling gives a significant decrease in movement restriction and muscle tension by which your acupuncture treatment can have a bigger profit, affecting the tissues at a deeper level.

ADDITIONAL INFORMATION REGARDING DIVING-RELATED DISORDERS

Chinese Medicine
Neck and lower back disorders seen with divers are usually caused by overload (resulting in stagnation of Qi and Xue). They might be combined with emotional issues (e.g. stress, fear), a physical disorder (e.g. osteoarthritis) or an external factor (e.g. Bi-syndrome).

Note: Regarding the several patterns I will explain the actions of the acupuncture points together in one section as there are corresponding acupuncture points.

Pattern Differentiation
1 Overload (Stagnation of Qi and Xue)
Overload includes walking to the waterfront or climbing up the stairs to get on the boat wearing the heavy diving equipment (tank, weight belt or integrated weight pockets), too heavy or prolonged sports training or repetitive movements.

- Clinical Signs and Symptoms

    - Fixed pain and rigidity of the neck/lower back (decreased range of motion)
    - Tension in the muscles
    - Reduced mobility in the facet joint due to muscle tension or shifting/dislocation of the vertebrae
    - Radiation of pain to and tingling sensation in the extremities
    - There may be Ashi Points (including Trigger Points).

Pulse: Wiry (*Xian*) or Choppy (*Se*).

Tongue: No signs (in the initial stage), dark or purple (or with purple stasis spots).

- Treatment Principle

    – Promote the circulation of Qi and Xue.
    – Alleviate pain.
    – Benefit the muscles and facet joints.

- Acupuncture Points (select from)
LI-4 Hegu, **LIV-3** Taichong, **SP-10** Xuehai, **SI-3** Houxi, **BL-62** Shenmai, **KI-3** Taixi, **GV-4** Mingmen, **BL-23** Shenshu, **BL-10** Tianzhu, **GV-16** Fengfu, **GB-20** Fengchi, **GB-21** Jianjing, **BL-36** Chengfu, **BL-40** Weizhong, **BL-57** Chengsan, **BL-60** Kunlun, YNSA Basic A, B, C, D, D1–D6 and E Points, Huatuo Jiaji Points, Ashi Points, Ear Point: Shenmen.

2 Mechanical Trauma

A mechanical trauma like whiplash or a fall might result in the disposition of one or more vertebrae and hypertonic muscles, combined with Qi and Xue stagnation. When walking to the waterfront wearing the heavy diving equipment or walking back to the shore through the ocean waves the diver should be very careful not to fall as it may result in severe joint problems. Especially when making *night dives* (diving when the sun is down), the diver has more risk of falling when walking to or back from the waterfront, simply because it is dark.

● Clinical Signs and Symptoms

- Muscle tension (often as a result of a disturbed coordination from the intrinsic muscles due to the mechanical forces)
- Fixed pain and/or radiation of pain to and tingling sensation in the extremities
- Disposition of vertebrae and reduced mobility in the facet joint due to muscle tension or shifting/dislocation of the vertebrae
- Decreased range of motion
- There may be Ashi Points (including Trigger Points)
- Emotional disbalance may be present.

Pulse: Wiry (*Xian*) or Choppy (*Se*).

Tongue: No signs (in the initial stage), dark or purple (or with purple stasis spots).

● Treatment Principle

— Promote the circulation of Qi and Xue.

— Alleviate pain.

— Benefit the muscles and facet joints.

● Acupuncture Points (select from)

LI-4 Hegu, **LIV-3** Taichong, **SP-10** Xuehai, **SI-3** Houxi, **BL-62** Shenmai, **KI-3** Taixi, **GV-4** Mingmen, **BL-23** Shenshu, **BL-10** Tianzhu, **GV-16** Fengfu, **GB-20** Fengchi, **GB-21** Jianjing, **BL-36** Chengfu, **BL-40** Weizhong, **BL-57** Chengsan, **BL-60** Kunlun, YNSA Basic A, B, C, D, D1–D6 and E Points, Huatuo Jiaji Points, Ashi Points, Ear Point: Shenmen.

3 Bi-Syndrome (Painful Obstruction Syndrome)

External pathogens such as Wind, Cold, Heat and Dampness can invade the body separately or in combination, causing various types of Bi-syndrome.

ADDITIONAL INFORMATION REGARDING DIVING-RELATED DISORDERS

This is especially likely when the body is weak, the external pathogen strong, or exposure to the external pathogen protracted. External pathogens obstruct the circulation of Qi and Xue in the channels, resulting in joint, muscle and sinew pain. Wind-Cold and Wind-Heat often attack the neck and upper part of the back, Wind-Dampness more the lower back.

Diving in colder water without sufficient body protection (e.g. no hood or a too thin diving suit) or when wearing wet swimwear for too long enables Cold-Dampness to invade the body. It's important not to sweat before diving as it will open the pores and makes the body more sensitive to an invasion of external Cold-Dampness (even when diving in tropical oceans/seas the water gets colder in the depths). In a tropical surrounding it is recommended to put on the diving suit just before entering the water to prevent sweating by getting too warm.

There are also divers who make *ice dives* (diving under ice) and they wear special dry suits to protect themselves against the cold, but hypothermia is still one of the risks.

- Clinical Signs and Symptoms

    - Pain and stiffness of the neck/lower back
    - Wind causes pain that migrates
    - Severe and fixed pain in the case of Cold
    - Heaviness and fixed pain in the case of Dampness
    - Burning pain when there is Heat
    - Swollen joints (in particular in the case of Dampness and Heat)
    - Muscle tension and possibly reduced mobility in the facet joints, decreased range of motion
    - Radiation of pain to and tingling sensation in the extremities.

Pulse:

- External Wind: Floating (*Fu*).
- External Cold: Tight (*Jin*), Slow (*Chi*).
- External Heat: Rapid (*Shuo*).
- External Dampness: Soggy (*Ru*).

Tongue:

- External Cold: normal (in the initial stage) or with a thin white coating.
- External Heat: normal (in the initial stage) or with a red front or a thin yellow coating.

- External Dampness: normal (in the initial stage) or with a greasy, white or yellow coating.

● Treatment Principle
- Expel Wind, Cold, Heat and/or Dampness.
- Alleviate pain.
- Benefit the muscles and facet joints.

● Acupuncture Points (select from)
BL-10 Tianzhu, **GV-16** Fengfu, **GB-20** Fengchi, **GB-21** Jianjing, **SP-9** Yinlingquan, **LI-11** Quchi, **LI-4** Hegu, **SI-3** Houxi, **BL-62** Shenmai, **GV-4** Mingmen, **BL-23** Shenshu, YNSA Basic A, B, C, D, D1–D6 and E Points, Huatuo Jiaji Points, Ashi Points, Ear Point: Shenmen.

4 Kidney Deficiency (Yin, Yang, Jing)
Doing too much for a long time, not enough rest, hormonal issues, too much physical exercise, excessive sexual activity, loss of Jin Ye and/or Xue, or having recently recovered from a chronic disease may weaken the lower back.

● Clinical Signs and Symptoms
- Mild but protracted pain, decreased range of motion
- Starts subtly
- Weakness in the lower back
- Cold feeling in the lower back and knees (Yang deficiency)
- Tiredness around 5 p.m.

Pulse:
- Kidney-Yin deficiency: Thready (*Xi*) and Rapid (*Shuo*).
- Kidney-Yang deficiency: Deep (*Chen*), Thready (*Xi*) and Slow (*Chi*).
- Kidney-Jing deficiency: Deep (*Chen*), Thready (*Xi*) and Weak (*Ruo*).

Tongue:
- Kidney-Yin deficiency: Red and dry with a slight, yellow or no coating.
- Kidney-Yang deficiency: Pale and white coating.
- Kidney-Jing deficiency: Variable to more Yin or Yang deficiency.

ADDITIONAL INFORMATION REGARDING DIVING-RELATED DISORDERS

- Treatment Principle
  - Nourish and tonify Kidney-Yin, Kidney-Yang and/or Kidney-Jing.
  - Alleviate pain.
  - Benefit the muscles and facet joints.

- Acupuncture Points (select from)
  KI-3 Taixi, **KI-6** Zhaohai, **CV-4** Guanyuan, **CV-6** Qihai, **GV-4** Mingmen, **BL-23** Shenshu, **SI-3** Houxi, **BL-62** Shenmai, **BL-10** Tianzhu, **GV-16** Fengfu, **GB-20** Fengchi, **GB-21** Jiangjing, **BL-36** Chengfu, **BL-40** Weizhong, **BL-57** Chengsan, **BL-60** Kunlun, YNSA Basic A, B, C, D, D1–D6 and E Points, Huatuo Jiaji Points, Ashi Points, Ear Point: Shenmen.

- Explanation: Neck and Back Disorders
  - **LI-4**–**LIV-3** combination promotes the free flow of Qi and Xue.
  - **SP-10** moves Qi.
  - **SI-3**–**BL-62** combination (Opening Points Du Mai) opens the Qi of the spine.
  - **KI-3**, **KI-6**, **CV-4**, **CV-6**, **GV-4** and **BL-23** nourish and tonify the Kidney, strengthen/benefit the lumbar spine (for their different actions see Table 1.7.5).
    - Use moxa in the case of Kidney-Yang and Kidney-Jing deficiency.
  - **BL-10**, **GV-16** and **GB-20** expel Wind, benefit the neck and alleviate occipital muscle tension.
  - **GB-21** relaxes the trapezius muscle.
  - **BL-36**, **BL-40**, **BL-57** and **BL-60** can be used in the case of radiating sensations in the legs.
  - **SP-9** is recommended in the case of Dampness, **LI-11** to clear Heat and **LI-4** to expel external Wind and to regulate Wei-Qi.
  - YNSA Basic A Point benefits the cervical spine (see Figure 1.7.3).
  - YNSA Basic B Point benefits the cervical spine and shoulder area (neck–shoulder–arm syndrome).
  - YNSA basic C Point benefits the upper extremities (in e.g. paraesthesia).
  - YNSA Basic D Point and D1–D6 Point benefit the lumbar spine, sacrum and coccyx.

- YNSA Basic E Point benefits the thoracic spine.

- Huatuo Jiaji Points from the most fixed vertebral segments improve the mobility and reduce muscle tension of the facet joints (see 'Clinical Notes' in Section 1.12.4A).

- Ashi Points (including Trigger Points) alleviate pain and muscle tension.

- Ear Point: Shenmen alleviates pain.

- Moxa can be used to expel Cold in the case of Wind-Cold, Kidney-Yang and Kidney-Jing deficiency.

● Clinical Notes

- Extraordinary vessel Du Mai: Du Mai is the symbol of the Yang energy, it is the Sea of Yang and connects with all Yang channels. Du Mai stands for mental and physical power and communication with the outside world. Deficiency of Du Mai leads to kyphosis of the spine and a lack of mental strength. Fullness of Du Mai results in hyperextension of the spine combined with pain and stiffness.

    Opening Points Du Mai: Master Point **SI-3** Houxi combined with Couple Point **BL-62** Shenmai. They open the Qi of the spine, strengthen the back and legs, relieve radiation of pain into the legs. Opening Du Mai is very effective for all neck and back disorders, headaches and migraines. Du Mai connects the spine with the brain and supports Kidney-Yang and Kidney-Jing.

- **Caution:** Don't needle **GV-16** deeply because the *medulla oblongata* is in the deep layer. Needle in between 0.5 and 1 CUN and in caudal direction (NOT cranial!). Destruction of the medulla oblongata is fatal because it's the origin of some important nerves of the body, which perceive sound and are instrumental in carrying on the function of breathing.

- I use the YNSA Basic D Point (Yin side) combined with Shenmen in the ear when a patient has too much pain in the lumbar zone to sit to do the intake or to lay down for the treatment. Usually after a few minutes the pain decreases so that further treatment is possible.

- When you treat someone at the front side of the body and there are spine problems as well, combining your acupuncture treatment with the YNSA Basic A, B, C, D, D1–D6 and/or E Points gives very good results. That's the way I prefer to use these points when there is a main issue that needs to be treated at the frontal side. In a treatment focused specifically on the neck or back itself I don't use the YNSA points but treat with Huatuo Jiaji points, Ashi points and **SI-3–BL-62** combination, **GB-20**, **GB-21**, and so on.

ADDITIONAL INFORMATION REGARDING DIVING-RELATED DISORDERS

- When you perform a (or a number of) mobilization technique(s) on the spinal column (e.g. oscillations of the lumbar spine) and/or a little massage before needling you can achieve quicker recovery.

● YNSA Basic Points

The YNSA basic points affect the kinetic apparatus. The YNSA basic points I use for spine disorders are the A, B, C, D, D1–D6 and E Points at the anterior (Yin) side of the head (see Figure 1.7.3). The details below are taken mainly from Yamamoto and Yamamoto's *Yamamoto New Scalp Acupuncture*.[2]

- The *Basic A Point* represents the head, cervical spine and those parts of the body supplied by nerves derived from this region.

    Location: Approximately 1 cm bilateral from the midline, at the hairline. The A Point is subdivided into A1–A8 following a vertical line from *inferior* to *superior* (with a total length of circa 2 cm). A3 (C3 nerve root) is at the hairline, A1 (C1 nerve root) is about 1 cm anterior to the hairline and A8 (C8 nerve root) is about 1 cm posterior to the hairline.

- The *Basic B Point* represents the cervical spine and areas innervated by the cervical nerves (shoulder and scapular region).

    Location: Approximately 1 cm bilateral to the Basic A Point, or 2 cm lateral to the midline, at the hairline.

- The *Basic C Point* represents the upper extremities and can be subdivided into nine smaller parts (C1–C9).

    Location: Approximately 2.5 cm lateral to the Basic B Point, or 4.5–5 cm bilateral to the midline. The Basic C Point is a line of about 2 cm length that runs in a direction of 45 degrees towards the root of the nose. The Basic C Point starts about 1 cm posterior to the hairline (shoulder) and ends about 1 cm anterior of the hairline (hand).

- The *Basic D Point* represents the lumbar spine and lower extremities.

    Location: Approximately 1 cm above the zygomatic arch, at the hairline, and 2 cm in front of the ear.

- The *D1–D6 Point* is a division of the Basic D point and represents the lumbar spine, sacrum and coccyx (D1–D5 = lumbar vertebrae 1–5; D6 = sacrum/coccyx).

    Location: A vertical line of about 1 cm and located above the TMJ region, just in front of the ear.

---

[2] Yamamoto, T. and Yamamoto, H., *Yamamoto New Scalp Acupuncture: YNSA*, Medical Tribune Inc., Tokyo, 2006.

DIVING MEDICAL ACUPUNCTURE

- The *Basic E Point* represents the thoracic spine, the ribs, thoracic cavity and internal organs innervated by the thoracic nerves.

  Location: Above the eyebrow, starting approximately 1 cm lateral to the midline (E12) and following a 15-degree oblique line laterally (total length about 2 cm) ending in E1.

● Food

To strengthen the Kidney and support the lower back the following foods are good: soups, beans, sea salt, seaweed and coconut water.

⬇ Advice for the Diver

- Take care that the tank is attached well to your BCD jacket. The tank should not touch your head.

- Your weight belt should be in the right position (should not give pressure in the lower back). Internal weight pockets may be very helpful.

- It's possible to avoid having the weight of the tank on your back at the surface by putting on your equipment in the water, providing there is not much current and there is time enough to join the other divers.

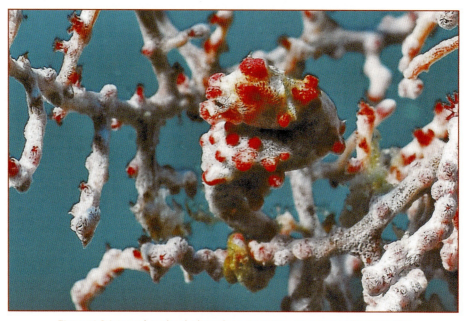

Figure 6.2.1 A neck or back disorder can cause severe problems under water. This tiny pygmy seahorse (1 cm long) is probably happy not needing to wear a heavy tank with compressed air on his back...
Photo: Janneke Vermeulen, Bohol Island, the Philippines, 2008

6.3 MUSCLE DISORDERS
肌肉的疾患

Muscle disorders seen with divers are mostly muscle cramps in the legs, especially the calves. Swimming against the current takes effort from the legs, and the calves can easily cramp while contracting in plantar flexion performed by the gastrocnemius and soleus muscles. The cold sea water can influence the blood circulation negatively. A wetsuit appropriate for the specific surrounding can help keeping the body as warm as possible (see 'Advice for the Diver' below). Avoiding dehydration is very important for preventing cramps and/or decompression illness.

Western Medicine
Definition and Aetiology
Muscle cramps are spontaneous painful contractions of muscle fibres due to heavy physical effort, lack of minerals (magnesium, calcium, zinc, salt, glucose), dehydration, cooling of the body, illness, intoxication, mechanical trauma.

Chinese Medicine
Pattern Differentiation

1. Stasis of Xue
2. Liver-Qi stagnation
3. Phlegm due to Spleen deficiency.

- Treatment Principle
  - Promote the circulation of Xue.
  - Spread Liver-Qi.
  - Transform Phlegm and tonify the Spleen.

- Acupuncture Points (select from)
  SP-10 Xuehai, **BL-17** Geshu, **BL-40** Weizhong, **LU-9** Taiyuan, **LI-4** Hegu, **LIV-3** Taichong, **PC-6** Neiguan, **BL-57** Chengshan, **ST-40** Fenglong, **SP-6** Sanyinjiao, **SP-4** Gongsun, **SP-3** Taibai.

- Explanation
  - **SP-10**, **BL-17** and **BL-40** move Xue.

- **LU-9** supports all blood circulation problems (e.g. cold hands and feet).
- **LI-4–LIV-3** combination and/or **PC-6** in Liver-Qi stagnation. **LI-4–LIV-3** combination also moves Xue.
- **BL-57** alleviates cramps in the calves.
- **ST-40** transforms Phlegm.
- **SP-6**, **SP-4** and **SP-3** tonify the Spleen to prevent the formation of Dampness and Phlegm.

● Food

- Cinnamon twig supports the blood circulation in the small capillaries.
- Magnesium relaxes the muscles.

Advice for the Diver

- Protect your body with a diving suit adequate for the area where you are going to dive. There are different kinds of suits: a tropical suit, which is just a thin neoprene layer; a wetsuit with several thicknesses (3 mm, for water 28–30 degrees Celsius, 5 mm for 20–27 degrees Celsius, and 7 mm for 3–19 degrees Celsius); and a dry suit for cold circumstances.
- Eat and drink properly so your glucose level will be okay and take care to take enough hydration.
- Take some extra vitamins and/or minerals when you are on a diving holiday because diving takes a lot of energy, especially when making many dives per day, making deep dives or drift dives (e.g. multivitamin or vitamin C and magnesium).
- Stretch your leg muscles before the dive.
- Don't dive when you are tired because you will get muscle cramps more easily (and, as said previously, there is more risk of decompression illness).
- Have a good night's sleep to prepare physically for diving, and to recover from previous dives if you dive on sequential days.

ADDITIONAL INFORMATION REGARDING DIVING-RELATED DISORDERS

6.4 LUNG DISORDERS
肺的疾患

Western Medicine

Under no circumstance may you dive if you have ever had a spontaneous pneumothorax or if you currently have asthma. If you only had asthma in early childhood and have had a recent virus or allergy that affected the lungs it might be possible to be examined fit for diving providing the lung function is okay again.

The cold and dry air from the regulator might trigger spasms in the bronchial system. Obstructions in the lungs can lead to air trapping. Air trapping means that air stays behind mucous in the bronchus or that the bronchus is obstructed itself. It can lead to barotrauma because there is no ventilation possible and alveoli can rupture when the ambient pressure changes. Prevent air trapping when an X-ray shows mucous in the lungs by solving the phlegm problem.

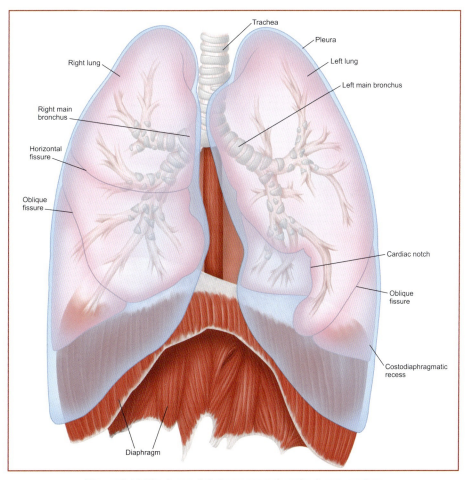

Figure 6.4.1 The lungs. It is important that the lungs are free of phlegm because its presence can lead to air trapping

You need well-functioning lungs for diving with an optimal elasticity, which can adapt to the changing ambient pressure. With certain lung disorders (e.g. bronchospasms, emphysema, phlegm) a diver will not be examined fit for diving because the lungs are air-containing and very vulnerable organs with a high risk of barotrauma in the case of pathology. When not functioning well there is a big risk of barotrauma (ruptured alveoli with arterial gas embolism as a result, pneumothorax leading to mediastinal emphysema or subcutaneous emphysema).

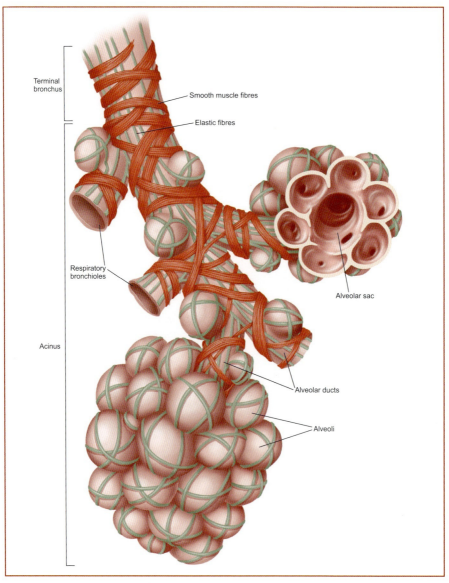

Figure 6.4.2 When the alveoli rupture due to overpressure, arterial gas embolism (AGE) can be a result

ADDITIONAL INFORMATION REGARDING DIVING-RELATED DISORDERS

Diagnosis
Use pulmonary function tests. An X-ray should be done with smokers to exclude air trapping.

Chinese Medicine
The focus here is on how to support the Lung and its function in general so divers will be able to inhale and exhale better and, if there is Phlegm, to transform that. When the Lung works better due to acupuncture the diver will be able to breathe more easy and deeply, which means the air tank gets empty less quickly! A diver will be grateful to you for every extra moment he or she can stay under water! When in poor condition the diver will consume lots of air whereby the tank will be empty very soon, resulting in a short dive.

- Treatment Principle
    - Fortify the Lung.
    - Promote the descending and diffusing of Lung-Qi.
    - Transform Phlegm.

- Acupuncture Points (select from)
LU-7 Lieque, **LU-9** Taiyuan, **BL-13** Feishu, **LU-2** Yunmen, **CV-17** Shanzhong, **ST-40** Fenglong, **SP-6** Sanyinjiao.

- Explanation
    - **LU-7**, **LU-9** and **BL-13** fortify the Lung and promote the descending and diffusing of Lung-Qi.
    - **LU-2** disseminates and descends Lung-Qi.
    - **CV-17** regulates Qi and unbinds the chest.
    - **ST-40** transforms Phlegm.
    - **SP-6** tonifies the Spleen to prevent the formation of Dampness and Phlegm.

- Food
    - Dry ginger builds Wei Qi, fresh ginger makes Phlegm more soft and relieves a cough.
    - Asparagus and honey feed the Lung-Yin.

- You can make tea from lily flowers to support the Lung-Qi.
- It is better to have no or little sugar and no cow's milk to prevent the formation of Phlegm.

⬇ Advice for the Diver

- If you have had lung problems, only dive after visiting a pulmonologist who is trained to test if you are fit to dive.
- It's better not to smoke when you are a diver because it diminishes the general condition and there is more risk of air trapping.
- Nicotine irritates the mucosa and stimulates the production of phlegm. The lungs are one of the most sensitive parts of the body when diving so extra care for them is needed!

6.5 HEART DISORDERS
心的疾患

In relation to the heart, in this book I focus only on whether you still are allowed to dive after myocardial infarction (heart attack) and on cardiac arrhythmia (irregular heartbeat). When having heart problems a diver always should be examined by a cardiologist to see if he or she is fit for diving or not.

Western Medicine
Treatment

- Beta-blockers
- ACE-inhibitors (angiotensin-converting-enzyme inhibitors)
- Anticoagulants (e.g. coumarins)
- Antiplatelets (e.g. aspirin)
- Paracetamol.

Caution: Beta-blockers lower the heart frequency, the blood pressure and the VO2 max. Lung oedema might be an effect. However, diving with beta-blockers is possible in some specific cases. After having had myocardial infarction a diver may dive again after one year and being examined fit for diving by a cardiologist specialized in diving medicine. An adequate effort tolerance has to be present.

ADDITIONAL INFORMATION REGARDING DIVING-RELATED DISORDERS

Diving after myocardial infarction with ACE-inhibitors is allowed if agreed by the examining cardiologist. The diver has to check – for example in a swimming pool – that the medication does not cause coughing under water.

Anticoagulants and antiplatelets can be absolute or relative contraindications for diving. Aspirin is safe to use but coumarins are absolutely contraindicated as they can cause bleeding in the spinal cord.

Lifestyle

It's important to work on a good condition, body weight and emotional balance after having had myocardial infarction. Some hospitals provide a sports programme accompanied by a doctor and/or physiotherapist. The programme is built up carefully and the patient is supervised to ensure exercises are performed well. When leaving the hospital it's necessary to keep on going with the changed lifestyle and work on good physical and mental health (walking, cycling, meditation, healthy food, not too much work pressure, etc.). Acupuncture is a good way to support general health.

Chinese Medicine

Myocardial infarction and cardiac arrhythmia frequently are the result of disturbed emotions. Emotional stress like anger blocks the Liver-Qi, which might suppress the Heart and cause stagnation of Heart-Xue (myocardial infarction) and/or deficiency of Heart-Yin or Heart-Qi (cardiac arrhythmia). Heart-Xue stasis can be caused by Heart-Yang deficiency as well (with underlying Spleen-Yang or Kidney-Yang deficiency), ending in Heart-Yang collapse (myocardial infarction). Phlegm can cause myocardial infarction as well by obstructing the Heart. Often there is fear about the heart disorder. It should be possible to recognize which pattern there has been before the infarction depending on how long after the trauma that the diver visits you for treatment. Focus on tonifying the presenting deficiency and/or promoting the flow of Qi and Xue.

Pattern Differentiation

1. Liver-Qi stagnation
2. Heart-Yin deficiency
3. Heart-Qi deficiency
4. Heart-Xue stasis
5. Heart-Yang deficiency ➔ Heart-Yang collapse
6. Phlegm obstruction.

- **Treatment Principle**
    - Spread Liver-Qi.
    - Nourish and tonify the Heart.
    - Promote the circulation of Heart-Xue.
    - Calm the Shen.

- **Acupuncture Points (select from)**

    LI-4 Hegu, **LIV-3** Taichong, **PC-6** Neiguan, **LIV-5** Ligou, **BL-15** Xinshu, **HT-5** Tongli, **HT-6** Yinxi, **HT-7** Shenmen, **HT-9** Shaochong, **BL-17** Geshu, **SP-10** Xuchai, **ST-40** Fenglong, **CV-17** Shanzhong, **M-HN-3** Yintang, Ear Point: Shenmen.

- **Explanation**
    - **LI-4–LIV-3** combination and **PC-6** spread Liver-Qi. **LI-4–LIV-3** combination moves Xue as well. **PC-6** also regulates the Heart and unbinds the chest.
    - **LIV-5** spreads the Liver-Qi and helps in plum-stone syndrome, which indicates unexpressed emotions.
    - **BL-15** nourishes the Heart and resolves stasis of Xue.
    - **HT-5** regulates the Heart rhythm.
    - **HT-6** regulates Heart-Xue.
    - **HT-7** regulates and tonifies the Heart besides calming the Shen.
    - **HT-9** regulates the Heart-Qi and revives consciousness.
    - **BL-17** and **SP-10** move Xue.
    - **ST-40** and **CV-17** transform Phlegm. **CV-17** unbinds the chest.
    - Yintang and Ear Point Shenmen calm the Shen.

- **Clinical Notes**
    - **HT-9** is an emergency heart attack point.
    - In the case of Heart-Yang deficiency/Heart-Yang collapse: support the underlying deficiency of Heart-Qi, Spleen-Yang and/or Kidney-Yang. In the case of Phlegm: support the Spleen.

ADDITIONAL INFORMATION REGARDING DIVING-RELATED DISORDERS

⬇ Advice for the Diver

After a heart attack:

- Only dive after having consulted a cardiologist and if any prescribed medication is no contraindication for diving.

- Work on a good physical and mental condition. Reduce stress and balance the emotions.

When having an irregular heartbeat:

- Don't make dives that can be stressful, such as deep dives, cave dives or drift dives.

- Not too much coffee, no rooibos tea or star mix tea. Rooibos and star mix tea can trigger irregular heartbeat. It is better to take green tea or fresh mint tea, which calms the Liver, or water with fresh lemon juice.

- Eat enough fruit and vegetables per day.

- Always take care of your general condition when you dive and rest well before diving (good sleep during the night and no physical exercises in between the dives on a diving holiday).

6.6 DIGESTIVE DISORDERS
消化疾患

Digestive disorders are not really diving related. Here I will restrict the subject by applying some advice regarding tropical infections, food and drinks to make diving more comfortable.

Check the blood and/or stools when you suspect a patient of having parasites, a Helicobacter or other pathogens. Divers who travel to tropical zones have a big chance of becoming infected with parasites, viruses, bacteria and fungi because people who live in the Western countries are not used to less clean situations (sanitary, food).

⬇ Advice for the Diver

- Don't eat heavy meals before diving.

- Don't drink carbonated beverages. The gas bubbles might give cramps in the intestines under water when the bubbles get larger.

- Don't drink too much coffee.

- Drink enough water before and after the dive to prevent dehydration (see 'Advice for the Diver' in Chapter 4).

- It's better not to drink alcohol during a diving holiday. In between the dives it's forbidden because it influences the reaction of the brain and under water the effect of alcohol is increased by the pressure of the water. In the evening after the dives it is better not to drink alcohol as well because it dehydrates the body, which has effects the day after.

- Don't swallow air while diving as air in the stomach will expand during the ascent.

6.7 STRESS AND PANIC
压力和惊慌

Western Medicine

Definition and Aetiology

Stress: Tension in body and mind.

Panic: State of fear.

Panic is the biggest cause of diving accidents (30–40%). Most diving accidents due to panic occur between a diver's 11th and 25th dive. People mostly ascend too quickly due to fear and panic (during an emergency ascent), ignorance of the laws of physics that apply to diving, and after bad dive instruction.

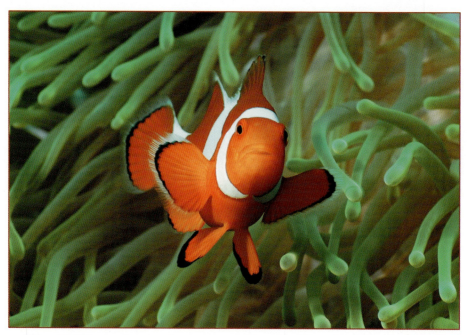

Figure 6.7.1 Famous Nemo, who swam away from the safe reef and brought himself trouble. Most diving accidents happen due to panic resulting from overconfidence
Photo: Janneke Vermeulen, Bohol Island, the Philippines, 2008

ADDITIONAL INFORMATION REGARDING DIVING-RELATED DISORDERS

People who are prone to stress, panic and hyperventilation may not be good candidates for diving. In the past people were mainly tested on physical issues but nowadays doctors also check psychological factors to see if a diver is capable of diving. In these cases diving might be discouraged. A quickly panicked diver can easily drown him or herself and be a danger for his or her buddy too.

Training is a good option to prevent panic because the diver then gets used to a specific situation or new diving equipment, or is able to perform a certain diving skill better.

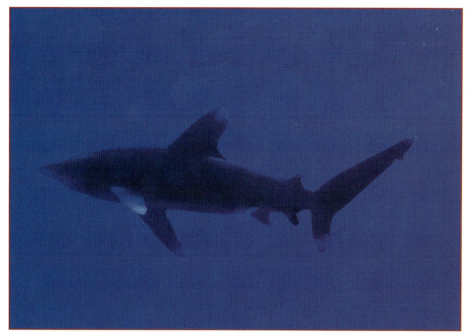

Figure 6.7.2 This white-tip shark is the first shark I photographed and I was yelling under water from happiness, not knowing I would have to push the shark away with my underwater housing a couple of minutes later... When I saw the teeth of the shark at 0.5 m distance, I knew I had to do something and pushed the underwater housing against his nose – not hard, but clear enough that the shark would think, 'This is not eatable.' I did stay calm but in the night I saw the shark's face coming in my direction 100 times...
Photo: Janneke Vermeulen, Red Sea, Egypt, 2008

Treatment

Medication for stress:

- Beta-blockers
- Antidepressants (tricyclic and SSRI)
- Benzodiazepines.

Medication for fear and panic:

- MAO inhibitors
- Antidepressants (tricyclic and SSRI)
- Benzodiazepines.

All these medications have lots of side-effects like decreased exercise tolerance or sedation, which can lead to severe problems under water.

Chinese Medicine
Pattern Differentiation
1 Liver-Qi Stagnation

Stress disrupts the circulation of Liver-Qi. When the Liver-Qi stagnates people don't feel well in general. They may have clinical signs and symptoms like sighing, hiccups, *plum-stone syndrome* (feeling as if they have a plum stone in the throat) or Phlegm retaining in the throat, all contributing to an uncomfortable condition while diving. Having stress when diving is risky as it influences your judgement and responsiveness negatively.

Pulse: Wiry (*Xian*).

Tongue: No signs or dark.

● Treatment Principle

- Spread Liver-Qi.
- Calm the Shen.

● Acupuncture Points (select from)
LI-4 Hegu, **LIV-3** Taichong, **PC-6** Neiguan, **LIV-5** Ligou, **GV-24** Shenting, **HT-7** Shenmen, Ear Points: Shenmen and Sympathetic Autonomic Point.

● Explanation

- **LI-4–LIV-3** combination and **PC-6** spread Liver-Qi.
- **LIV-5** spreads the Liver-Qi and helps in plum-stone syndrome (which indicates unexpressed emotions).
- **GV-24** calms the Liver and Shen.
- **HT-7** and Ear Point Shenmen calm the Shen.
- Ear Point: Sympathetic Autonomic Point calms the sympathetic autonomic system, which is overstimulated in stress and panic.

ADDITIONAL INFORMATION REGARDING DIVING-RELATED DISORDERS

2 Kidney Deficiency

The Kidney is related to fear, which can deplete the Kidney. A sudden fright descends Kidney-Qi by blocking the Upper Jiao (Upper Burner) and long-term fear ascends the Qi and may affect the Heart (a strong Heart and fear result in descending of Qi, a weak Heart and fear in ascending of Qi).[3] Kidney deficiency itself can also lead to fear. With fear related to Kidney deficiency there may be clinical signs and symptoms like frequent urination, pain in the lower back, weakness of the knees, dizziness and tinnitus. When people cannot cope with fear it can result in panic and for divers that is very dangerous as it may result in a too rapid ascent to get back to the water surface.

Pulse:

- Kidney-Yin deficiency: Thready (*Xi*) and Rapid (*Shuo*).
- Kidney-Yang deficiency: Deep (*Chen*), Thready (*Xi*) and Slow (*Chi*).
- Kidney-Jing deficiency: Deep (*Chen*), Thready (*Xi*) and Weak (*Ruo*).

Tongue:

- Kidney-Yin deficiency: Red and dry with a slight, yellow or no coating.
- Kidney-Yang deficiency: Pale and a white coating.
- Kidney-Jing deficiency: Variable to more Yin or Yang deficiency.

● Treatment Principle

- Raise Qi.
- Nourish and tonify Kidney-Yin, Kidney-Yang and/or Kidney-Jing.

● Acupuncture Points (select from)

GV-20 Baihui, **HT-7** Shenmen, **KI-1** Yongquan, **KI-3** Taixi, **KI-6** Zhaohai, **CV-4** Guanyuan, **CV-6** Qihai, **GV-4** Mingmen, **BL-23** Shenshu.

● Explanation

- **GV-20** and **HT-7** calm the Shen. **GV-20** raises Yang-Qi.
- **KI-1**, **KI-3**, **KI-6**, **CV-4**, **CV-6**, **GV-4** and **BL-23** nourish and tonify the Kidney (for their different actions see Table 1.7.5).
    - Use moxa in the case of Kidney-Yang and Kidney-Jing deficiency.

---

3 Maciocia, G., *The Psyche in Chinese Medicine*, Churchill Livingstone Elsevier, London, 2009.

- Clinical Notes
    - In the case of fear, Maciocia (2009) advises unblocking the Upper Jiao with **HT-5** Tongli and **LU-7** Lieque (besides raising the Qi with **GV-20**).[4]

- Food

Soups, beans, sea salt and seaweed strengthen the Kidney.

- Lifestyle

Take enough physical rest to recover.

Advice for the Diver

- Use relaxation techniques like meditation and listening to calming music to increase a general feeling of relaxation in daily life.

- Take time to get used to new equipment or a new surrounding. You need to know how new equipment works before you dive with it. Diving requires your full attention, and being busy with your equipment distracts you from necessary diving actions (like checking your air, the bottom time, the depth, the surrounding and monitoring your buddy).

- A clear *briefing* before every dive is very important. It can easily give stress when it is not clear what the dive will be like.

    Note: For non-divers it is not well known that a briefing is common before every dive. A briefing means that the whole dive will be discussed before going under water. When a diver is at a diving resort or at a live-a-board the Divemaster who accompanies the dive will make a simple drawing on a board of the underwater surroundings where the dive will take place. He or she will mark the maximum depth and the bottom time. He or she will tell you what you can expect to see under water (e.g. turtles, sharks) and how the surrounding looks (e.g. corals), warn you of certain things like a *washing machine* (also known as a kolk) or a down current, and tell you where you start, turn and end the dive. You may agree on, for instance, what the halfway point of the dive will be (it's the point where you turn in direction of the starting point of the dive or where you decide to start ascending). It could be a mark in the surroundings or when having 100 ATA compressed air left in the tank. Another common agreement in diving concerns the moment there is 50 ATA air left in the tank. In that case you always start ascending to the

---

4 Maciocia, G., *The Psyche in Chinese Medicine*, Churchill Livingstone Elsevier, London, 2009.

water surface and have your three-minute safety stop at the 5-metre level before you end the dive.

- Dives should be prepared very well, and even more so when the dives include more danger like cave diving or technical diving[5] or, for example, descending to 100 metres below the water surface. When people are easily stressed cave diving and technical diving should be discouraged.

- Make sure you have good communication with your buddy-diver.

- It is better not to drink coffee before diving if you are very susceptible to stress. Caffeine leads to the release of adrenalin, which can aggravate the feelings of stress.

- If you are susceptible to hyperventilation you probably should not dive. It might mean that you can have stress reactions more quickly which can be very dangerous when under water.

- To prevent an accident, you must not dive when under acute stress.

---

5 According to PADI *technical diving* implies going beyond recreational scuba diving limits, for example going deeper than 40 metres, dives that require staged decompression (stopping at set depths and times during final stages of ascent for off-gassing), using variable gas mixtures during the dive, or using extensive equipment.

CHAPTER 7

DIVING AND MEDITATION
潜水与冥想

7.1 INTRODUCTION

Being under water is mysterious and that's why the waterspirit mermaid has been used in many stories, like Walt Disney's version, and in myths and sagas in the past. In ancient Chinese stories the mermaid is seen as a force in nature which symbolizes power and mystics, and when she cries her tears can change into pearls. Celtic sagas talk about the mermaid as the symbol of medical knowledge: she swam to the shore to give advice to people on how to cure diseases. In Caribbean myths the mermaid Siren protects all that lives in the ocean.

7.2 MEDITATION AND FLOTATION
冥想与漂浮

Going down under the water surface and entering another world calms the mind and can have the same effect as meditation. Diving is associated with the Water Element, one of the Five Elements that are the basis of Chinese medicine. The Water Element is associated with the Kidney and according to Bridges (2012) the primary physical healing actions of the Kidney relate to being, meditating and finding spirituality; its healing emotions are wisdom and allowing.[1]

Daoism principles like Yin and Yang become even more clear when in the magic underwater world. The mass of the water is Yin and the movements of it are Yang. There is oneness. You feel one with nature. The feeling of time and space disappears and you feel free. A one-hour dive feels like 20 minutes. There is the feeling of only you, the sound of the bubbles from the regulator and a fairytale surrounding with wonderful colours and corals, many different-shaped fish, sea turtles, sharks, manta rays and sparkling sunbeams reflecting in the water. Creation is happening in this timeless space. Things become clear and ideas come into your mind. How is that possible?

---

1   Bridges, L.P., *Face Reading in Chinese Medicine*, second edition, Churchill Livingstone, Elsevier, London, 2012.

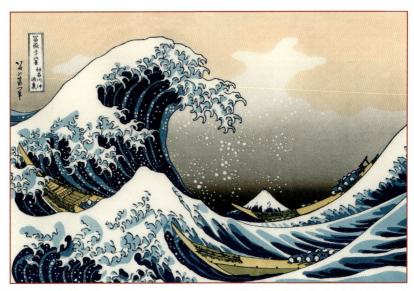

Figure 7.2.1 'The Great Wave off Kanagawa' (1829–1833) by Katsushika Hokusai. The large wave expresses a massive Yin force to the Yang of empty space under it
Copyright Rijksmuseum Amsterdam, the Netherlands. Image from awesome-art.biz

A Western scientific explanation for getting insights, ideas and entrance to our creativity is based on brain chemistry that occurs in certain circumstances like meditation, sleeping and flotation. When we dive and regulate our buoyancy well, we *float* and it is likely that we encounter this specific brain activity.

7.3 FLOTATION TANK
漂浮罐

In 1954 an American neuroscientist, John C. Lilly, used floating for a new therapy. He invented a flotation tank to stimulate the brain and discovered that floating gave deep relaxation by activating *theta waves* combined with a very conscious mind.[2]

In the tank people were isolated from all external stimuli and Epsom salts was added into the water so the person could float. This, also called a *sensory deprivation tank,* is still used for meditation, relaxation and as integrated medicine by athletes in Australia to recover more quickly after exercising.[3] Another name for this method is *floating REST*: restricted environmental stimulation therapy.

Experiments in flotation tanks have shown the following effects, whereby we may conclude that theta waves are important for healing:

---

2   Lilly, J.C., 'The John C. Lilly Homepage', http://johnclilly.com (accessed 14 August 2017).
3   Semerda, E.W., 'Floatation: Sensory Deprivation for Engineers by Scientists' [blog post], The Road to Silicon Valley, 10 July 2012, www.theroadtosiliconvalley.com/local-california/floatation-tank-isolation-tanks (accessed 14 August 2017).

- reduction of stress, anxiety and depression
- better sleep
- decrease in perception of pain (in e.g. chronic stress-related pain, fibromyalgia)
- increase in optimistic feelings and the content of the vitalizing hormone prolactin[4]
- reduction of hypertension, muscle tension and levels of cortisol
- improvement in well-being and performance (lowering of stress during perceptual motor coordination)
- possible practical use for burnout and chronic fatigue.[5]

7.4 BRAIN WAVES
脑电波

When diving we are not in a restricted environment like a flotation tank but the floating aspect is there and sounds are very limited. When floating and being weightless, theta waves in the cerebral cortex are especially active. The brain is relaxed and drowsy in this state (subconscious level). Theta waves have a low frequency (4–8 Hz), are present during the REM part of sleep and are the most active just before we awake and before falling asleep: when there is a change from subconsciousness to consciousness and vice versa.

Psychologist and expert in brain wave patterns Anna Wise wrote (2002), 'Theta provides the subconscious, inner information and wisdom. In its pure form, this is not experienced with clear imagery, rather having hazy, dream-like qualities of deep internal reverie.'[6] Creativity can occur in this state.

Alpha waves (8–16 Hz) are also active at these relaxed moments and they are the 'link between the conscious and subconscious mind'.[7] Alpha waves make it possible for the information from the theta waves to be processed and interpreted at a *beta* level (16–32 Hz). It is due to the stimulation of alpha waves that we can remember our dreams and images clearly. Alpha activity is the portal to meditation.[8]

While diving you have to be alert and beta waves, which are produced by our thinking mind, are active too. Thinking is needed during a dive because you

---

4 Swedish Research Council, 'Floating effective for stress and pain, research suggests', *Science Daily*, 6 November 2006.
5 Dierendonck, D. van and Nijenhuis, J. te, 'Flotation restricted environmental stimulation therapy (REST) as a stress-management tool: A meta-analysis', *Psychology and Health* 2005, 20, 3, 405–412.
6 Wise, A., *Awakening the Mind*, Jeremy P. Tarcher/Putnam, New York, 2002 (p.140).
7 Wise, A., *Awakening the Mind*, Jeremy P. Tarcher/Putnam, New York, 2002 (p.11).
8 Wise, A., *Awakening the Mind*, Jeremy P. Tarcher/Putnam, New York, 2002.

have to be aware of yourself, your surrounding, your equipment (air, depth, etc.) and you have to anticipate what may happen. Beta waves are related to creative thinking but also to anxiety, panic and an overactive mind, and can be stimulated by drinking coffee.

Being in a theta state is an important condition when wanting to meditate at an unconsciousness *delta* level (1–4 Hz), which is the deepest state of meditation and occurs during sleep. In some people delta waves can be active when they are awake. They work as 'unconscious scanning' and involve our intuition, empathy, instinct and inner knowing. Delta waves are usually manifest in medical professionals.[9] When you have profound medical knowledge your intuition can guide you as you have the skills and tools to examine if what your inside is telling you is right. Activating theta waves during flotation may also support the medical professional to have easier access to this delta level.

Regardless, the beneficial changes in brain chemistry that occur while floating can cause a general feeling of well-being and balance in the diver.

When you descend under the water surface you become part of the world of mermaids and mermen. You leave behind your daily life and enter into an underwater landscape of extraordinary impressions. In this silent universe your thoughts – quiet as your awareness – are absorbed in the pervading stillness. You become present in the moment, with clarity and focus, and are able to access your creative mind without the inner monologue. Once you have visited this magical space you don't forget it and you want to go back without any hesitation.

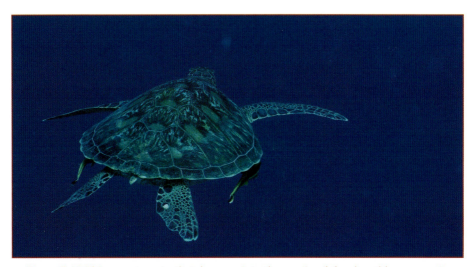

Figure 7.4.1 This green sea turtle takes you into the magic of the deep blue ocean. In Chinese medicine the turtle stands for wisdom and longevity. This seems very appropriate given the turtle's life of floating and the theta waves it must experience!
Photo: Janneke Vermeulen, Bohol Island, the Philippines, 2008

---

9   Wise, A., *Awakening the Mind*, Jeremy P. Tarcher/Putnam, New York, 2002.

CONCLUSION

With this work I hope I have made obvious how you can help divers when they are not fit to dive. It is important to know what kind of consequences can come from being submerged and to have profound knowledge about diving medicine and Chinese medicine.

When you are aware of what happens below the water surface, it is possible to treat and support lots of physical and mental disorders of divers and make diving a great experience again. The divers will be very grateful for your treatment!

Maybe you are even triggered now to get your own diving licence. Doing that will extend your knowledge and insights about this subject even more, and having your own experiences under water will bring to life how it is to be a part of the underwater world!

Besides this I hope this book contributes to more understanding about ENT and TMJ disorders in general and that the offered information will trigger you to look more deeply into these subjects.

APPENDIX I

Glossary of Terminology

Table AI.1 Vital substances

Gu Qi	Food Qi
Jing	Essence (the clearest distillation of essence)
Jin Ye	Body Fluids
Shen	Spirit (all emotional, mental and spiritual energies of a person)
Wei Qi	Defensive or Protective Qi
Xue	Blood
Ying Qi	Nutritive Qi
Zong Qi	Gathering Qi

Table AI.2 Channel abbreviations

LU	Lung
LI	Large Intestine
ST	Stomach
SP	Spleen
HT	Heart
SI	Small Intestine
BL	Bladder
KI	Kidney
PC	Pericard
TB	Triple Burner
GB	Gall Bladder
LIV	Liver
CV	Conception Vessel
GV	Governing Vessel

Table AI.3 Pulse qualities

Choppy	Se
Deep	Chen
Deficient	Xu
Floating	Fu
Full	Shi
Rapid	Shuo
Slippery	Hua
Slow	Chi
Soggy	Ru
Thready	Xi
Tight	Jin
Weak	Ruo
Wiry	Xian

APPENDIX II

Acupuncture Points with Specific ENT and TMJ Actions

LUNG CHANNEL

LU-2 Yunmen *Cloud Gate*
Actions: Disseminates and descends Lung-Qi.

LU-5 Chize *Cubit Marsh*
Actions: Clears Lung-Heat, descends rebellious Qi.

LU-7 Lieque *Broken Sequence*
Actions: Expels Wind-Cold, Wind-Heat, releases the exterior, fortifies Lung-Qi, nourishes Lung-Yin (when combined with **KI-6**[1]), promotes the descending and diffusing of Lung-Qi, benefits the nose, throat, head and neck.

LU-9 Taiyuan *Supreme Abyss*
Actions: Tonifies Lung-Qi, nourishes Lung-Yin, promotes the descending of Lung-Qi (which prevents Jin Ye stagnating in the nose and sinuses), transforms Phlegm.

LU-10 Yuji *Fish Border*
Actions: Clears Lung-Heat, descends rebellious Qi, benefits the throat.

LU-11 Shaoshang *Lesser Shang*
Actions: Expels Wind-Heat, benefits the throat.

LARGE INTESTINE CHANNEL

LI-4 Hegu *Joining Valley*
Actions: Expels Wind-Cold, Wind-Heat, releases the exterior, regulates Wei Qi, adjusts sweating, promotes the diffusing of Lung-Qi, restores the Yang, benefits the nose, sinuses, throat, ears and head.

LI-11 Quchi *Pool at the Crook*
Actions: Eliminates Wind, clears Heat, releases the exterior, benefits the throat, supports immunity.

LI-20 Yingxiang *Welcome Fragrance*
Actions: Expels Wind, clears Heat, opens the nose and maxillary sinus.

STOMACH CHANNEL

ST-2 Sibai *Four Whites*
Actions: Eliminates Wind, clears Heat, benefits the maxillary sinus and the eyes.

ST-3 Juliao *Great Crevice*
Actions: Eliminates Wind, dissipates pain and swelling of the nose, cheek and lips, alleviates pain in the maxillary sinus.

ST-6 Jiache *Jaw Bone*
Actions: Alleviates pain, benefits the TMJ (improves the range of motion in the TMJ, alleviates tension/spasm of the masseter muscle).

---

1   Maciocia, G., *De Grondslagen van de Chinese Geneeskunde, Een Complete Basishandleiding voor Acupuncturisten en Fytotherapeuten, Tweede Uitgave*, Churchill Livingstone, New York, 2005.

ST-7 Xiaguan *Below the Joint*
Actions: Expels Wind, alleviates pain, benefits the TMJ and ears.

ST-25 Tianshu *Heaven's Pivot*
Actions: Resolves Dampness and Damp-Heat, regulates the Spleen, Stomach and intestines, eliminates stagnation from the abdomen, calms the Shen.

ST-36 Zusanli *Leg Three Miles*
Actions: Tonifies Qi, fortifies the Spleen, resolves Dampness and Phlegm, supports the immune system.

ST-40 Fenglong *Abundant Bulge*
Actions: Transforms Phlegm and Dampness.

ST-44 Neiting *Inner Courtyard*
Actions: Clears Heat from the Stomach channel, benefits the throat, ears and TMJ.

SPLEEN CHANNEL

SP-3 Taibai *Supreme White*
Actions: Tonifies the Spleen, resolves Dampness and Damp-Heat.

SP-4 Gongsun *Grandfather Grandson*
Actions: Fortifies the Spleen, resolves Dampness, calms the Shen.

SP-6 Sanyinjiao *Three Yin Intersection*
Actions: Tonifies the Spleen, resolves Dampness, spreads the Liver-Qi, harmonizes the Liver, supports general tonification (Qi, Yin and Xue) and immunity.

SP-9 Yinlingquan *Yin Mound Spring*
Actions: Resolves Dampness and regulates the Spleen.

SP-10 Xuehai *Sea of Blood*
Actions: Invigorates Xue and dispels stasis.

HEART CHANNEL

HT-7 Shenmen *Spirit Gate*
Actions: Regulates and tonifies the Heart, calms the Shen.

SMALL INTESTINE CHANNEL

SI-3 Houxi *Back Stream*
Actions: Clears Wind-Heat, benefits the ears.

SI-17 Tianrong *Heavenly Appearance*
Actions: Benefits the ears, throat and TMJ (relaxes muscles and tendons).

SI-19 Tinggong *Palace of Hearing*
Actions: Eliminates Wind, clears Heat, benefits the ears, improves hearing acuity, benefits the TMJ, calms the Shen.

BLADDER CHANNEL

BL-2 Zanzhu *Gathered Bamboo*
Actions: Expels Wind, clears the nose and frontal sinuses, benefits the eyes.

BL-10 Tianzhu *Celestial Pillar*
Actions: Regulates Qi, expels Wind, alleviates pain, relieves occipital tension (relaxes muscles and tendons), benefits the head.

BL-12 Fengmen *Wind Gate*
Actions: Expels Wind, releases the exterior, strengthens Wei Qi, promotes the descending and diffusing of Lung-Qi, benefits the nose.

BL-13 Feishu *Lung Shu*
Actions: Tonifies Lung-Qi, nourishes Lung-Yin, releases the exterior, promotes the descending and diffusing of Lung-Qi.

BL-17 Geshu *Diaphragm Shu*
Actions: Invigorates Xue and dispels stasis, cools Xue and stops bleeding, nourishes and harmonizes Xue, benefits the sinews.

BL-18 Ganshu *Liver Shu*
Actions: Spreads Liver-Qi, regulates and nourishes Liver-Xue, cools Fire and clears Damp-Heat, stabilizes the Shen, benefits the eyes and sinews.

BL-20 Pishu *Spleen Shu*
Actions: Tonifies the Spleen, resolves Dampness and nourishes Xue.

ACUPUNCTURE POINTS WITH SPECIFIC ENT AND TMJ ACTIONS

BL-23 Shenshu *Kidney Shu*
Actions: Nourishes Kidney-Yin, fortifies Kidney-Yang and benefits Kidney-Jing, the eyes and ears.

BL-62 Shenmai *Extending Vessel*
Actions: Expels Wind, subdues rebellious Qi from the head, calms the Shen, benefits the head and eyes.

KIDNEY CHANNEL

KI-1 Yongquan *Gushing Spring*
Actions: Descends excess from the head, nourishes Kidney-Yin, calms the Shen.

KI-3 Taixi *Supreme Stream*
Actions: Nourishes Kidney-Yin, tonifies Kidney-Yang, clears deficiency Heat, benefits the Lung, head, throat and ears.

KI-6 Zhaohai *Shining Sea*
Actions: Nourishes Kidney-Yin and Jin Ye, clears deficiency Heat, benefits the throat.

KI-27 Shufu *Shu Mansion*
Actions: Spreads and descends Lung-Qi.

PERICARD CHANNEL

PC-6 Neiguan *Inner Pass*
Actions: Spreads the Liver-Qi, calms the Shen, harmonizes the Stomach, alleviates nausea and vomiting, clears Heat, affects the vestibular organ and the nervous system.

TRIPLE BURNER CHANNEL

TB-2 Yemen *Fluid Gate*
Actions: Clears Heat in the Triple Burner, calms the Shen, benefits the ears.

TB-3 Zhongzhu *Central Islet*
Actions: Expels Wind, clears Heat in the head, subdues Liver-Yang, benefits the ears.

TB-5 Waiguan *Outer Pass*
Actions: Expels Wind-Cold, Wind-Heat, Wind-Damp, releases the exterior, subdues Liver-Yang, benefits the head, neck, eyes and ears.

TB-17 Yifeng *Wind Screen*
Actions: Eliminates Wind, clears Heat, benefits the ears, improves hearing acuity, activates the channel and alleviates pain.

TB-21 Ermen *Ear Gate*
Actions: Eliminates Wind, clears Heat, benefits the ears, improves hearing acuity.

GALL BLADDER CHANNEL

GB-2 Tinghui *Meeting of Hearing*
Actions: Eliminates Wind, clears Heat, benefits the ears, improves hearing acuity, benefits the TMJ, activates the channel and alleviates pain.

GB-8 Shuaigu *Leading Valley*
Actions: Subdues Liver-Yang, treats intoxications (alcohol, coffee, nicotine), benefits the head, alleviates pain.

GB-14 Yangbai *Yang White*
Actions: Subdues Liver-Yang, eliminates Wind, benefits the head and eyes and alleviates pain.

GB-20 Fengchi *Wind Pool*
Actions: Eliminates Wind, subdues Liver-Yang, benefits the head (occiput), neck, nose, throat and ears.

GB-21 Jiangjing *Shoulder Well*
Actions: Regulates Qi, alleviates pain, relaxes the tendons and muscles (neck region, especially trapezius muscle).

GB-34 Yanglingquan *Yang Mound Spring*
Actions: Clears Damp-Heat in the Liver-Gall Bladder, spreads Liver-Qi, benefits the sinews and joints.

GB-39 Xuanzong *Suspended Bell*
Actions: Promotes the free flow of the Liver-Qi, clears Gall Bladder Fire.

GB-42 Diwuhui *Earth Five Meetings*
Actions: Spreads Liver-Qi and clears Gall Bladder-Heat, benefits the ears, improves hearing.

GB-43 Xiaxi *Clamped Stream*
Actions: Clears Damp-Heat from the Gall Bladder channel, clears Heat, benefits the head and ears.

LIVER CHANNEL

LIV-2 Xingjian *Moving Between*
Actions: Clears Liver-Fire, subdues Liver-Yang, spreads Liver-Qi.

LIV-3 Taichong *Great Rushing*
Actions: Spreads Liver-Qi and Xue, nourishes Liver-Yin, subdues Liver-Yang, clears Liver-Fire, calms the Shen and spasms, resolves muscle contractions, muscle tension and pain.

LIV-5 Ligou *Woodworm Canal*
Actions: Spreads Liver-Qi, treats plum-stone syndrome.

LIV-8 Ququan *Spring at the Crook*
Actions: Tonifies Liver-Yin and Xue, subdues Liver-Yang.

CONCEPTION CHANNEL

CV-4 Guanyuan *Gate of Origin*
Actions: Tonifies and nourishes Kidney-Yin, Kidney-Yang, Kidney-Jing, fortifies Qi, Yin, Yang and Xue in general.

CV-6 Qihai *Sea of Qi*
Actions: Tonifies Kidney-Yang and fortifies Qi in general.

CV-12 Zhongwan *Middle Cavity*
Actions: Fortifies the Spleen, resolves Dampness and Phlegm.

CV-17 Shanzhong *Chest Centre*
Actions: Regulates Qi, unbinds the chest, descends rebellious Lung-Qi, clears the Lung and transforms Phlegm.

GOVERNING CHANNEL

GV-4 Mingmen *Gate of Life*
Actions: Tonifies the Kidney, regulates especially Kidney-Yang, clears Heat.

GV-14 Dazhui *Great Vertebra*
Actions: Expels Wind, firms the exterior, clears Heat.

GV-16 Fengfu *Palace of Wind*
Actions: Expels Wind, nourishes the Sea of Marrow, benefits the head and neck, calms the mind.

GV-20 Baihui *Hundred Meetings*
Actions: Subdues Liver-Yang, nourishes the Sea of Marrow, benefits the head, calms the Shen.

GV-23 Shangxing *Upper Star*
Actions: Eliminates Wind, dispels swelling and benefits the head, face, eyes and nose.

EXTRA POINTS

M-HN-3 Yintang *Hall of Impression*
Actions: Expels Wind, benefits the nose and frontal sinuses, calms the Shen.

M-HN-6 Yuyao *Fish Waist*
Actions: Benefits the forehead, eye, eyelid and frontal sinus.

M-HN-9 Taiyang *Sun (Supreme Yang)*
Actions: Eliminates Wind, clears Heat, benefits the frontal and maxillary sinus, relaxes the temporalis muscle and affects the trigeminal nerve.

M-HN-14 Bitong, also called Shangyingxiang *Penetrating the Nose*
Actions: Benefits the nose and maxillary sinus.

(EX) Biyan *Eyes of Nose*
Actions: Benefits the nose.

YAMAMOTO NEW SCALP ACUPUNCTURE (YNSA)

Eye Point
Actions: Benefits the eyes.

Nose Point
Actions: Benefits the nose.

Mouth Point
Actions: Benefits the mouth.

Ear Point
Actions: Benefits the ears and TMJ.

TMJ Point
Actions: Benefits the TMJ.

Basic A Point
Actions: Benefits the cervical spine.

ACUPUNCTURE POINTS WITH SPECIFIC ENT AND TMJ ACTIONS

WRIST ACUPUNCTURE

Wrist Point 1 (Upper 1)
  Actions: Benefits the nose and throat.

Wrist Point 4 (Upper 4)
  Actions: Benefits the ears and TMJ.

Vertigo and Auditory Zone
  Actions: Benefits the ears.

EAR ACUPUNCTURE

Inner Ear.C
  Actions: Benefits the ears.

Inner Ear.E
  Actions: Benefits the ears.

Shenmen
  Actions: Calms the Shen, alleviates pain.

TMJ
  Actions: Benefits the TMJ in general.

APPENDIX III

Acupuncture Points with Specific ENT- and TMJ- Related Indications

LUNG CHANNEL

LU-2 Yunmen *Cloud Gate*
Indications: Cough, wheezing, dyspnoea.

LU-5 Chize *Cubit Marsh*
Indications: Cough, coughing up phlegm, wheezing, dyspnoea, pain and swelling in the throat, dry mouth and tongue.

LU-7 Lieque *Broken Sequence*
Indications: Cough, coughing up phlegm, wheezing, dyspnoea, nasal congestion and discharge, nasal polyp, pain and swelling in the throat, stiff neck, fever, chills.

LU-9 Taiyuan *Supreme Abyss*
Indications: Cough, cough with phlegm, wheezing, dyspnoea.

LU-10 Yuji *Fish Border*
Indications: Pain and swelling in the throat, dry throat, cough, dyspnoea, heat in the body. This point is very effective when having no voice – after needling the voice can return in one day.

LU-11 Shaoshang *Lesser Shang*
Indications: Pain and swelling in the throat, cough, dyspnoea, swollen tonsils, fever. In the case of an extremely sore throat/laryngitis you can perform a blood-letting technique on **LU-11** to reduce the Heat.

LARGE INTESTINE CHANNEL

LI-4 Hegu *Joining Valley*
Indications: Nasal congestion and discharge, sneezing, sinus disorders, pain and swelling in the throat, loss of voice, deafness, tinnitus, headache (especially frontal headache), fever, chills, aversion to cold, sweating or absence of sweating.

LI-11 Quchi *Pool at the Crook*
Indications: Pain and swelling in the throat, loss of voice, fever, thirst.

LI-20 Yingxiang *Welcome Fragrance*
Indications: Nasal congestion and discharge, sneezing, anosmia, nasal polyp, maxillary sinusitis (pain, swelling, phlegm).

STOMACH CHANNEL

ST-2 Sibai *Four Whites*
Indications: Redness, pain and itching of the eyes, lacrimation, headache.

ST-3 Juliao *Great Crevice*
Indications: Maxillary sinusitis (pain, swelling, phlegm).

ST-6 Jiache *Jaw Bone*
Indications: TMJ disorders (inability to chew, pain and tension/spasm in the masseter muscle), stiffness and pain of the neck, loss of voice, parotitis (e.g. mumps).

ACUPUNCTURE POINTS WITH SPECIFIC ENT- AND TMJ-RELATED INDICATIONS

ST-7 Xiaguan *Below the Joint*
Indications: Tinnitus, deafness, ear pain, itching and purulent discharge from the ear, trigeminal neuralgia, TMJ disorders (pain, tension, arthritis, dislocation, luxation).

ST-25 Tianshu *Heaven's Pivot*
Indications: Vomiting, retching, seasickness, motion sickness, stress, fear.

ST-36 Zusanli *Leg Three Miles*
Indications: Tiredness, fever, chills, aversion to cold, pain and swelling in the throat with inability to speak, headache, dizziness, tinnitus, palpitations, immune enhancement, general tonification, nausea, vomiting, epigastric pain, hiccups.

ST-40 Fenglong *Abundant Bulge*
Indications: Copious phlegm, cough, wheezing, dyspnoea, swelling and pain in the throat, plum-stone syndrome, headache, Wind-Phlegm headache, heaviness of the body.

ST-44 Neiting *Inner Courtyard*
Indications: Heat in the head, pain and swelling in the throat, nosebleed, sinus pain, trigeminal neuralgia, thirst, tinnitus, seasickness, motion sickness, aversion to the sound of people speaking, longing for silence.

SPLEEN CHANNEL

SP-3 Taibai *Supreme White*
Indications: Heavy feeling in the head or body, undigested food in stools, constipation, abdominal pain and distension.

SP-4 Gongsun *Grandfather Grandson*
Indications: Fear, mental restlessness, insomnia, poor appetite, loose stools, borborygmus, nausea.

SP-6 Sanyinjiao *Three Yin Intersection*
Indications: Recurring or chronic ENT disorders (combined with disturbed emotions, in particular overthinking), immunity enhancement, general tonification, tinnitus, dizziness, tiredness, palpitations.

SP-9 Yinlingquan *Yin Mound Spring*
Indications: Heaviness of the body and head, not clear thinking (foggy head), poor appetite.

HEART CHANNEL

HT-7 Shenmen *Spirit Gate*
Indications: Pain and swelling in the throat, dry throat with no desire to drink, stress, fear, worries.

SMALL INTESTINE CHANNEL

SI-3 Houxi *Back Stream*
Indications: Deafness, tinnitus, otitis, headache, dizziness, stiffness and pain of the neck.

SI-17 Tianrong *Celestial Countenance*
Indications: TMJ disorders, bruxism, tinnitus, deafness, parotitis, tonsillitis, pain and swelling in the throat, cough, wheezing, dyspnoea, chills, fever.

SI-19 Tinggong *Palace of Hearing*
Indications: Purulent discharge from the ear, ear pain, itching in the ear, deafness, tinnitus, blocked ears, tension in the jaw muscles.

BLADDER CHANNEL

BL-2 Zanzhu *Gathered Bamboo*
Indications: Nasal congestion and discharge, sneezing, anosmia, lacrimation, itching of the eyes, frontal headache, frontal sinusitis (pain, swelling, phlegm).

BL-10 Tianzhu *Celestial Pillar*
Indications: Nasal congestion, anosmia, lacrimation, swelling of the throat with difficulty speaking, (occipital) headache, stiff neck with inability to turn the head, dizziness, fever, aversion to cold.

BL-12 Fengmen *Wind Gate*
Indications: Cough, nasal congestion and discharge, sneezing, dyspnoea, fever, aversion to cold, occipital headache, stiff neck.

BL-13 Feishu *Lung Shu*
   Indications: Cough, coughing up phlegm, dyspnoea, cough or dyspnoea with pain in the upper back, pain and swelling in the throat, fever, chills, absence of sweating.

BL-17 Geshu *Diaphragm Shu*
   Indications: Nosebleed, cough, dyspnoea, throat painful obstruction.

BL-23 Shenshu *Kidney Shu*
   Indications: Tinnitus, dizziness, headache.

BL-62 Shenmai *Extending Vessel*
   Indications: Stiffness of the neck, (occipital) headache, dizziness, fever, chills, aversion to cold, aversion to wind with spontaneous sweating and headache, tinnitus, deafness, nosebleed, red eyes and eye pain.

KIDNEY CHANNEL

KI-1 Yongquan *Gushing Spring*
   Indications: Tinnitus.

KI-3 Taixi *Supreme Stream*
   Indications: Wheezing, dry cough, sore throat, dyspnoea, deafness, tinnitus, dizziness, headache.

KI-6 Zhaohai *Shining Sea*
   Indications: Pain, swelling, redness and dryness in the throat, dry cough, plum-stone syndrome.

KI-27 Shufu *Shu Mansion*
   Indications: Cough, wheezing, dyspnoea.

PERICARD CHANNEL

PC-6 Neiguan *Inner Pass*
   Indications: Nausea, vomiting, stress, fear, seasickness, motion sickness.

TRIPLE BURNER CHANNEL

TB-2 Yemen *Fluid Gate*
   Indications: Deafness, sudden deafness, tinnitus, ear pain.

TB-3 Zhongzhu *Central Islet*
   Indications: Ear pain, otitis media, deafness, tinnitus, dizziness, (temporal) headache, fever, chills, aversion to wind and cold, painful obstruction in the throat, blockage of the ears (especially useful when flying or after a flight).

TB-5 Waiguan *Outer Pass*
   Indications: Headache, stiff neck, fever, chills, aversion to cold, lacrimation due to wind and cold, ear pain, deafness, hearing loss, tinnitus, itching of the ear, redness, pain and swelling of the ear.

TB-17 Yifeng *Wind Screen*
   Indications: Tinnitus, deafness, ear discharge, ear ache, itching on the inside of the ear, redness, pain and swelling of the ear.

TB-21 Ermen *Ear Gate*
   Indications: Ear pain, tinnitus, deafness, itching, purulent discharge from the ear, redness and swelling of the ear.

GALL BLADDER CHANNEL

GB-2 Tinghui *Meeting of Hearing*
   Indications: Ear pain, purulent discharge from the ear, redness and swelling of the ear, itching of the ear, deafness, tinnitus (cricket sound), TMD (arthritis, luxation, pain, difficulty in masticating), parotitis.

GB-8 Shuaigu *Leading Valley*
   Indications: Intoxications (alcohol, coffee, nicotine).

GB-14 Yangbai *Yang White*
   Indications: Frontal headache, frontal sinusitis, lacrimation due to Wind.

GB-20 Fengchi *Wind Pool*
   Indications: Headache, stiff and painful neck (occipital), fever, chills, cold with absence of sweating, lacrimation due to wind, nasal congestion and discharge, rhinitis, nosebleed, pain and swelling of the throat, deafness, tinnitus, blocked ears.

ACUPUNCTURE POINTS WITH SPECIFIC ENT- AND TMJ-RELATED INDICATIONS

GB-21 Jianjing *Shoulder Well*
Indications: Cough, dyspnoea, stiffness and pain of the neck (trapezius muscle), TMJ disorders.

GB-34 Yanglingquan *Yang Mound Spring*
Indications: Bitter taste in the mouth, fever, dry throat, contractions of the sinews, stiffness and tightness of the muscles and joints, spasms.

GB-39 Xuanzong *Suspended Bell*
Indications: Dry mucosa in the nose, headache, stiff neck, dizziness, painful obstruction in the throat, nosebleed.

GB-42 Diwuhui *Earth Five Meetings*
Indications: Deafness, tinnitus.

GB-43 Xiaxi *Clamped Stream*
Indications: Headache, dizziness, pain and swelling of the cheek and submandibular region, deafness, tinnitus, itching in the ears, ear pain, otitis media, redness and pain of the outer canthus.

LIVER CHANNEL

LIV-2 Xingjian *Moving Between*
Indications: Bitter taste in the mouth, red eyes, thirst, cough, headache, dizziness, tinnitus.

LIV-3 Taichong *Great Rushing*
Indications: Distension and pain in the head and throat, headache, dizziness, tinnitus, insomnia, irritability.

LIV-5 Ligou *Woodworm Canal*
Indications: Plum-stone syndrome.

LIV-8 Ququan *Spring at the Crook*
Indications: Nosebleed, allergies of the respiratory tract, dry nasal mucous membranes.

CONCEPTION CHANNEL

CV-4 Guanyuan *Gate of Origin*
Indications: Dizziness, tinnitus, cough, dyspnoea.

CV-6 Qihai *Sea of Qi*
Indications: Deficiency of general body energy, tiredness, weak voice.

CV-12 Zhongwan *Middle Cavity*
Indications: Postnasal drip.

CV-17 Shanzhong *Chest Centre*
Indications: Useful when there is a tendency to getting the common cold quickly, tiredness, spontaneous sweating, weak voice, cough, wheezing, dyspnoea, phlegm, pain and fullness of the chest.

GOVERNING CHANNEL

GV-4 Ming Men *Gate of Life*
Indications: Tinnitus, dizziness.

GV-14 Dazhui *Great Vertebra*
Indications: Fever, chills, pain and swelling in the throat.

GV-16 Fengfu *Palace of Wind*
Indications: Aversion to cold, fever, body aches, stiffness and pain of the neck, occipital stiffness, headache, blurred vision, dizziness, tinnitus, nosebleed, painful obstruction throat and sudden loss of voice.

GV-20 Baihui *Hundred Meetings*
Indications: Tinnitus, dizziness, headache, nasal congestion and discharge, nosebleed.

GV-23 Shangxing *Upper Star*
Indications: Nasal congestion and discharge, sneezing, anosmia, nosebleed, nasal polyps, frontal and maxillary sinusitis.

EXTRA POINTS

M-HN-3 Yintang *Hall of Impression*
Indications: Nasal congestion and discharge, sneezing, anosmia, frontal headache, frontal sinusitis (pain, swelling, phlegm).

M-HN-6 Yuyao *Fish Waist*
Indications: Frontal headache, frontal sinusitis (pain, swelling and phlegm), puffy eyelids, lacrimation, itching and redness of the eyes, allergic conjunctivitis.

(EX) Biyan *Eyes of Nose*
Indications: Nasal congestion and discharge, anosmia. Especially effective in case of dryness of the mucosa due to long-term Liver-Qi stagnation/Liver Gall Bladder Fire.

M-HN-14 Bitong, also called Shangyingxiang *Penetrating the Nose*
Indications: Nasal congestion and discharge, maxillary sinusitis (pain, swelling and phlegm), lacrimation, clogged tear duct.

M-HN-9 Taiyang *Sun (Supreme Yang)*
Indications: Frontal and maxillary sinusitis (pain, swelling and phlegm), one-sided headache, dizziness, tinnitus, trigeminal neuralgia, bruxism, tension in the temporalis muscle.

WRIST POINTS

Wrist Point 1 (Upper 1)
Indications: Nasal congestion and discharge, anosmia, pharyngitis, tonsillitis, cough, chills, fever.

Wrist Point 4 (Upper 4)
Indications: Ear pain, tinnitus, hearing loss, TMJ disorders.

CHINESE SCALP ACUPUNCTURE

Vertigo and Auditory Zone Scalp
Indications: Tinnitus, deafness, loss of hearing, dizziness.

YAMAMOTO NEW SCALP ACUPUNCTURE (YNSA)

Eye Point
Indications: Conjunctivitis, lacrimation, dryness and pain of the eyes.

Nose Point
Indications: Nasal congestion and discharge, anosmia, sneezing, dryness of the mucosa in the nose, polyp.

Mouth Point
Indications: Tonsillitis, pharyngitis and TMJ pain.

Ear Point
Indications: Tinnitus, ear pain.

TMJ Point
Indications: TMJ disorders (arthritis, osteoarthritis, pain, muscle tension, dislocation), bruxism.

Basic A Point
Indications: Neck disorders.

EAR ACUPUNCTURE

Inner Ear.C
Indications: Tinnitus.

Inner Ear.E
Indications: Tinnitus.

Shenmen
Indications: Stress, muscle tension, tinnitus.

TMJ
Indications: TMJ disorders (arthritis, osteoarthritis, pain, muscle tension, dislocation), bruxism.